More Praise for *100 Questions & Answers About Vascular Anomalies*

"What an informative primer on vascular anomalies that Dr. Francine Blei has developed for the patient and their families. The question and answer format is indeed a most effective medium for making medical information available to the public. Dr. Blei has certainly chosen the relevant questions and has answered them in a simple, yet informative, manner. There is no doubt that the informed patient makes for a more satisfying and rewarding doctor-patient relationship. All of us who treat patients with vascular anomalies would agree with this statement. The text should also serve as a model to be developed in all areas of medicine. There is so much helpful and worthwhile information resulting from 100 Questions!"

Joseph G. McCarthy, MD
Lawrence D. Bell Professor of Plastic Surgery and Director,
The Institute of Reconstructive Plastic Surgery
NYU Langone Medical Center

"This book will be very beneficial to patients and families. Although most clinics use teaching information, this book accurately combines all of the information is an accurate, easy-to-read format. We will use this as a teaching tool in our clinic."

Denise Adams, MD
Medical Director of the Hemangioma and
Vascular Malformations Center
Cincinnati Children's Hospital

D1605671

"Dr. Francine Blei (a physician specializing in vascular anomalies) and Lita Anglin (a family health librarian who has a vascular malformation) have given us a most needed easy-to-read book on vascular anomalies in an organized, clear, comprehensive, and understandable format, for parents and patients with vascular anomalies—which are often very frightening, and frequently disfiguring, lesions. Their systematic approach is useful not only for patients and their families, but to healthcare professionals not familiar with vascular anomalies. Blei and Anglin identified the 100 most frequently asked questions encountered by those affected by this complex group of lesions, answering them in a professional but easily understood manner. We thank and congratulate the authors for this much needed book, which will rapidly become *a must!!* for our patients and their families."

Alejandro Berenstein, MD
Professor of Radiology and Neurosurgery
Albert Einstein School of Medicine
Co-Director of the Vascular Birthmark Institute of New York
Director of the Hyman Newman Institute of Neurology
and Neurosurgery, Roosevelt Hospital
New York, NY

"Adults and parents of children, who suffer from vascular anomalies, will find *100 Questions & Answers About Vascular Anomalies* to be an invaluable resource. Those affected with vascular anomalies often face multifaceted problems of cosmetic issues and chronic pain, as well as the difficulty of finding physicians who are knowledgeable about the field of vascular anomalies. Dr. Francine Blei and Ms. Lita Anglin have answers for questions about this little-understood area of medicine, and can point patients who suffer from vascular anomalies in the right direction toward finding the help and answers they need to find competent care."

Judy Vessey
Director
Klippel Trenaunay Support Group

"This easy-to-read and timely book has comprehensive questions that provide the answers we all seek during our journey with the care and treatment of a loved one living with a vascular anomaly. In very informative and understandable explanations, the family will be comforted learning more about their child's condition so they can be an effective advocate. The healthcare provider will be appreciative for a resource that saves valuable time in the office visit to focus on the patient and their family."

Karen L. Ball
President and CEO
The Sturge-Weber Foundation

"As I read the pages I keep thinking about how I wish I had access to this book 15 years ago. As a parent of a child with a hemangioma, this would have been a lifeline. As a patient advocate, it will be an invaluable resource guide to every person that contacts NOVA. When my daughter was first diagnosed with a hemangioma, I had many questions, but no one to provide me with answers. This book uniquely answers all those questions—in simple terms every parent can understand. Parents are told their infant has a birthmark, but in the following sentences words like hemangioma, tumor, anomaly, and malformation are used interchangeably. This book breaks down the complex medical terms so that every parent can learn exactly what their child has been diagnosed with and how it can be treated."

Karla Hall
Executive Director of the National Organization of Vascular Anomalies
(NOVA)

"Patients with vascular anomalies and their families often must resort to finding information on their own. Much of the medical and lay literature is confusing and commonly ill informed. With *100 Questions & Answers About Vascular Anomalies*, Dr. Blei simplifies the field for patients who frequently have difficulty finding accurate and reliable information. The references to additional credible sources for more detailed information will assist patients in their deeper quest to understand their specific conditions and find appropriate solutions."

Steven Fishman, MD
Stuart and Jane Weitzman Family Chair in Surgery
Co-Director, Vascular Anomalies Center
Children's Hospital, Boston
Harvard Medical School
Boston, MA

"Dr. Francine Blei is without question one of the world's foremost authorities on vascular anomalies, and this book is a must for any parent—and doctor—confronted with hemangiomas, port wine stains, and other vascular conditions. As a parent of a child who has dealt with such issues, I found this book to be both refreshing and informative."

Nicholas Sparks
Author of The Notebook *&* Message in a Bottle

"As a family advocate for the Vascular Birthmark Foundation, I found this book to be a valuable resource in helping families find clear and correct information on hemangiomas and vascular malformations. This comprehensive resource not only includes medical descriptions and answers, but patient/family support information and resources as well. Thank you, Dr. Blei, for your dedication to this field."

Corinne Barinaga
Vascular Birthmark Foundation Director of Family Services
MSN VB Support Group Manager

"This text is an invaluable resource for parents, patients, and doctors about the often misunderstood world of vascular anomalies . . . that affect so many children and families in need of support!"

Hannah Storm
ESPN Anchor

"As a family affected by a vascular birthmark, we've learned so much from this book! Dr. Francine Blei has written an essential, practical resource guide, based on her extensive experience researching and treating various types of vascular anomalies. Readers will find straightforward answers to questions regarding everything from proper diagnosis to the red flags and risks associated with these common, yet misunderstood, conditions. Dr. Blei's book will empower parents by providing them with the basic knowledge necessary to make educated decisions regarding their child's future course of treatment and overall well-being."

Donna and Evan Ducker
Co-Authors, *Buddy Booby's Birthmark*

"Patients with vascular anomalies face many challenges. Their diseases threaten physical appearance, function, and even survival. Among the many challenges faced by these patients and their families is the fact that it is often difficult, if not impossible, to find answers to their fundamental questions. Here, at last, is a concise and valuable resource that is destined to become a cornerstone in the pragmatic literature consulted both by patients and healthcare providers."

Stanley G. Rockson, MD
Allan and Tina Neill Professor of Lymphatic Research and Medicine
Director, Stanford Center for Lymphatic and Venous Disorders
Stanford University School of Medicine
Stanford, CA

"When our first baby was born, we just wanted her to be healthy. But when she was just 5 weeks old, we noticed an unusual bump growing underneath her eyelid. Soon we found out it was something called a hemangioma. World-renowned specialist Dr. Francine Blei provided us with the guidance we desperately needed to help us make it through a very difficult year. Would our daughter need to take steroids? Would her vision be altered? What would we say to onlookers who asked us what was wrong with her? In her book, *100 Questions & Answers About Vascular Anomalies*, Dr. Blei gives many other families the hope and comfort they will also need when faced with the unexpected consequences of dealing with a vascular anomaly."

Gretchen Carlson
Co-Host, Fox and Friends

"Having spent the past thirty years treating children and adults with vascular anomalies, I am pleased and impressed with the unique resource this book represents. Distilled into 100 succinct questions and answers, this volume covers virtually everything a patient or family needs to know. This contribution is particularly valuable in an area where there is so much confusion and misinformation even among medical practitioners. I recommend it without reservation."

Robert J. Rosen, MD
Director of Peripheral Vascular Intervention
Lenox Hill Heart and Vascular Institute
Director of Peripheral Vascular Intervention
Vascular Birthmark Institute of New York
New York, NY

"Dr. Francine Blei's book answers every conceivable question parents might have about their child's condition, treatment options, etiology, psychosocial issues, and resources. The book describes the wide range of vascular anomalies and, while not talking down to the reader, clarifies the characteristics of each condition. The glossary is easy and helpful for parents and others to use when they hear unfamiliar terms. A craniofacial malformation, or facial difference, can cause alarm, shame, anger, and depression in the parent. With this vast array of information, a parent, armed with full under-standing of the conditions, can be confident in the choices they make for their child. That is the great gift of this book."

Whitney Burnett
Executive Director
National Foundation for Facial Reconstruction
New York, NY

100 Questions & Answers About Vascular Anomalies

Francine Blei, MD, MBA
Professor of Pediatrics and Surgery (Plastic)
Medical Director, Vascular Anomalies Program
Institute of Reconstructvie Plastic Surgery and
Stephen D. Hassenfeld Center for Children with
Cancer and Blood Disorders
NYU Langone Medical Center
New York, New York

Carlita Anglin, MSIS
Family Health Librarian
Stephen D. Hassenfeld Center for Children
with Cancer and Blood Disorders
NYU Langone Medical Center
New York, New York

JONES AND BARTLETT PUBLISHERS
Sudbury, Massachusetts
BOSTON   TORONTO   LONDON   SINGAPORE

World Headquarters
Jones and Bartlett Publishers
40 Tall Pine Drive
Sudbury, MA 01776
978-443-5000
info@jbpub.com
www.jbpub.com

Jones and Bartlett Publishers
Canada
6339 Ormindale Way
Mississauga, Ontario L5V 1J2
Canada

Jones and Bartlett Publishers
International
Barb House, Barb Mews
London W6 7PA
United Kingdom

Jones and Bartlett's books and products are available through most bookstores and online book-sellers. To contact Jones and Bartlett Publishers directly, call 800-832-0034, fax 978-443-8000, or visit our website, www.jbpub.com.

Substantial discounts on bulk quantities of Jones and Bartlett's publications are available to corporations, professional associations, and other qualified organizations. For details and specific discount information, contact the special sales department at Jones and Bartlett via the above contact information or send an email to specialsales@jbpub.com.

The authors, editor, and publisher have made every effort to provide accurate information. However, they are not responsible for errors, omissions, or for any outcomes related to the use of the contents of this book and take no responsibility for the use of the products and procedures described. Treatments and side effects described in this book may not be applicable to all people; likewise, some people may require a dose or experience a side effect that is not described herein. Drugs and medical devices are discussed that may have limited availability controlled by the Food and Drug Administration (FDA) for use only in a research study or clinical trial. Research, clinical practice, and government regulations often change the accepted standard in this field. When consideration is being given to use of any drug in the clinical setting, the healthcare provider or reader is responsible for determining FDA status of the drug, reading the package insert, and reviewing prescribing information for the most up-to-date recommendations on dose, precautions, and contraindications, and determining the appropriate usage for the product. This is especially important in the case of drugs that are new or seldom used.

Production Credits
Executive Publisher: Christopher Davis
Editorial Assistant: Sara Cameron
Production Editor: Daniel Stone
Senior Marketing Manager: Barb Bartoszek
Manufacturing and Inventory Control
   Supervisor: Amy Bacus
Composition: Glyph International
Printing and Binding: Malloy, Inc.

Cover Credits
Cover Design: Carolyn Downer
Image Credit: Top: © Junial Enterprises/
   ShutterStock, Inc.; Bottom Left:
   © Julie DeGuia/ShutterStock, Inc.; Bottom
   Right: © Andrew Lever/ShutterStock, Inc.
Cover Printing: Malloy, Inc.

Library of Congress Cataloging-in-Publication Data
Blei, Francine.
  100 questions and answers about vascular anomalies / Francine Blei,
Carlita Anglin.
     p. cm.
  Includes bibliographical references and index.
  ISBN 978-0-7637-6659-7 (alk. paper)
  1. Cardiovascular system—Diseases—Popular works. I. Anglin, Carlita.
II. Title. III. Title: One hundred questions and answers about vascular
anomalies.
  RC672.B54 2011
  616.1—dc22
                    2010002520

6048

Printed in the United States of America
14 13 12 11 10 10 9 8 7 6 5 4 3 2 1

Contents

Questions 1–19 introduce basic facts about vascular anomalies, their causes, and the diagnosis process:
- How do vascular anomalies affect a person's circulatory system?
- What causes vascular anomalies?
- What are some of the key tests used to identify, diagnose, and classify vascular malformations?

Questions 20–42 describe many aspects of vascular malformations, including prognosis, treatments, and related conditions caused by the condition:
- What is a vascular malformation?
- What are some of the syndromes related to vascular malformations?
- What are some medications used to treat patients with vascular malformations?

Questions 43–73 review important facts about hemangiomas, such as types, causes, treatment options, and risks associated with this condition:
- What are some of the different kinds of hemangiomas?
- Are certain people more likely to have hemangiomas?
- When is surgery recommended to treat hemangiomas, and what are the possible complications?
- The doctor wants to evaluate my child for PHACES. What is that?

Questions 74–81 explain the effects of lymphatic malformations and associated syndromes, as well as treatment options:
- What is a lymphatic malformation?
- What precautions should I be aware of regarding lymphatic malformations?
- What are some of the syndromes associated with lymphatic malformations?

How can you learn more about vascular anomalies if you don't know you have one? Many patients have stories of being shuffled from one specialist to another without having a coordinated approach to care. Patients often have trouble finding experienced specialists in their area to receive a proper diagnosis.

Vascular anomalies are an overlooked area of medicine. In fact, the diagnosis is often delayed or incorrect due to the lack of awareness and experience in many specialties. Fortunately, this trend is improving as professional meetings include, or focus on, the evaluation and management of vascular anomalies, as well as controversies and new research in this field.

This book, which is divided into five major categories, attempts to answer the most common questions asked by patients and their family members. The first section addresses basic questions that are universal to all types of vascular anomalies. The second, third, and fourth sections are devoted to the unique issues related to vascular malformations, hemangiomas, and lymphatic malformations. The final section addresses practical questions related to living with a vascular anomaly.

This book is not intended to be exhaustive or highly technical; rather, it is a well-intentioned attempt to guide consumers toward reliable resources and knowledge that can assist them in formulating their own questions. Managing the initial and ongoing care of a vascular anomaly can be enormously frustrating and stressful for patients and families. We hope this book is helpful in defining the disorders and in helping patients and their family members navigate the field.

We would like to thank the patients and family members who have provided the impetus for this book. We are also very grateful to our colleagues at the Vascular Anomalies Program at NYU Langone Medical Center and elsewhere, as well as the many foundations that provide invaluable information, resources, and support to patients and families.

Francine Blei, MD, MBA
Carlita Anglin, MSIS

PART ONE

The Basics

How do vascular anomalies affect a person's circulatory system?

What causes vascular anomalies?

What are some of the key tests used to identify, diagnose, and classify vascular malformations?

More . . .

1. What is the circulatory system?

The circulatory, or cardiovascular, system is a complex body system that transports oxygen, nutrition, and waste throughout the body (Figure 1). The circulatory system networks the heart, blood vessels, arteries, and lungs in order to move blood and lymphatic fluid within the body. The heart pumps oxygen-rich blood to the body through the arteries. Veins send blood back to the heart.

Embryo

Early stages of growth and develop- ment in utero.

The circulatory system develops very early in the human **embryo**, with the heartbeat starting at 4–5 weeks of gestation.

2. What is the role and function of arteries, veins, and capillaries?

The arteries, veins, and capillaries are responsible for transporting blood throughout the body (Figure 2). Their function can be described as follows:

- *Arteries* are muscular, elastic vessels that carry oxy- gen-rich blood out to the body. The arterial system pushes blood throughout the body and bears the highest circulatory pressures; arteries close to the skin produce a person's pulse.
- *Arterioles* are the smallest and final branches of arte- rial vessels that bring fresh blood to distant parts of the body and then transition into capillaries.
- *Capillaries* are tiny blood vessels that act as exchange agents. They allow oxygen and nutrients to move from the blood to the body tissues and waste to pass from tissues back to the blood to be carried away. Capillaries bridge arteries and veins and then drain into venules.
- *Venules* are the smallest veins that connect veins and capillaries.
- *Veins* are the blood vessels that bring oxygen-poor blood back to the heart.

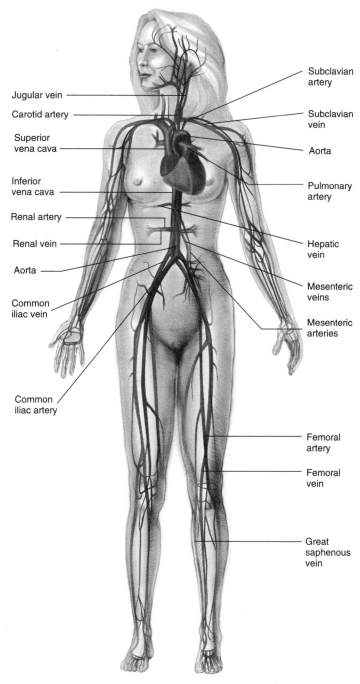

Figure 1   Circulatory system.

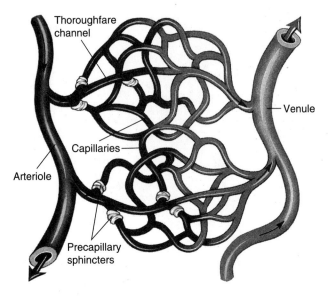

Figure 2   Network of veins and arteries.

3. What is the lymphatic system?

The lymphatic system is composed of lymph vessels, lymph nodes, and lymphatic ducts. Lymphatic fluid containing proteins, nutrients, and white blood cells (also called lymphocytes) circulate within lymphatic vessels. The lymphatic system helps maintain the body's balance of fluids, absorbs fats from the intestines to the bloodstream, and helps fight infections (Figure 3). Lymph nodes are a key part of the body's immune system, and they enlarge during certain infections or cancers. Jugular lymphatic trunks in the neck drain lymphatic fluids from both sides of the head and neck. The thoracic duct, the body's main lymphatic vessel, receives lymphatic fluid from the left jugular trunk and drains into the venous system. Lymphatic fluid is straw-colored; however it can appear "milky" after fat intake in lymphatics of the intestinal tract.

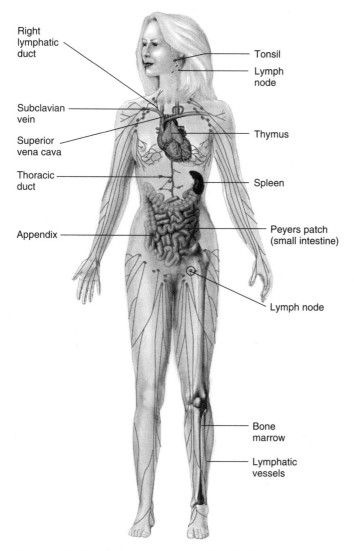

Right lymphatic duct

Tonsil

Lymph node

Subclavian vein

Superior vena cava

Thymus

Thoracic duct

Spleen

Appendix

Peyers patch (small intestine)

Lymph node

Bone marrow

Lymphatic vessels

Figure 3 **The lymphatic system consists of lymphatic vessels and ducts, lymph nodes (which are distributed throughout the body), the tonsils, the thymus gland, and the spleen.**

4. What are the key components of blood and lymphatics?

When discussing vascular anomalies, we are focusing on the blood and lymphatic vessels, which carry blood and lymphatic fluid. Blood vessels are the tubes through

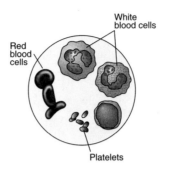

Figure 4   Components of blood.

which blood flows. Blood consists of cellular components as well as plasma, which perform many important functions. Lymphatic fluid plays an important role in fluid balance and infection control. Disorders of the cellular or plasma components of blood or lymphatic fluid can be associated with various disorders. Cellular components of the vascular (arterial/venous/capillary) system include white blood cells, red blood cells, and platelets (Figure 4). Red blood cells provide oxygen to tissues and exchange carbon dioxide for oxygen in the lungs, white blood cells help fight infection, and platelets help blood to clot. Plasma is the straw-colored fluid in which proteins (including coagulation factors), nutrients, and electrolytes (minerals) flow.

5. What are endothelial cells?

Endothelial cells are thin cells that make up the blood vessels and play an important role in the circulatory and lymphatic systems (Figure 5). Endothelial cells create a lining, the **endothelium**, inside heart and blood/lymphatic vessel walls. This special vessel lining improves the ability of blood components to be pumped farther and more efficiently throughout the body.

Endothelial cells

Cells that form blood vessels.

Endothelium

The thin layer of cells lining the interior surface of blood vessels.

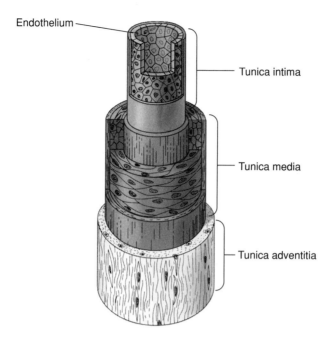

Endothelium

Tunica intima

Tunica media

Tunica adventitia

Figure 5   Endothelial cells.

Endothelial cells are involved in a number of key functions including:

- Vessel constriction and dilation
- Growth of new blood vessels (angiogenesis)
- Clotting
- Thickening of vessel walls
- Exchanges of gases and nutrients

In certain kinds of vascular anomalies such as hemangiomas, extra blood vessels are formed by a process called **angiogenesis**. These endothelial cells grow at a very fast rate over several months, termed the proliferative phase. The growth rate then stabilizes, and eventually the vascular mass spontaneously improves. This phase is called the involution stage.

Angiogenesis

Formation and development of new blood vessels.

The Basics

7

6. What is a vascular anomaly?

The term *vascular anomaly* refers to a wide range of disorders that vary in their presentation and medical seriousness. Although vascular anomalies are growths of vascular tissue and/or extra blood vessels, they are not cancerous. They are generally divided into two distinct categories based on their likelihood to grow:

1. *Static* (not growing)
2. *Proliferative* (growing during all or part of their life cycle)

A functional classification of the most common vascular anomalies follows (Figure 6):

In utero

In the uterus.

Gestation

Duration of growth of embryo and fetus before delivery. In humans full-term gestation is 40 weeks.

1. Those that are present **in utero** and grow in parallel with the growth of the patient are called *static vascular malformations* and can affect the capillaries, venules, veins, arteries, and lymphatics alone or in combination. These vessels have developed abnormally during **gestation**.

2. *Proliferative vascular lesions* grow disproportionately to the growth of a child, at least during part of his or

Proliferative Vascular Lesions (likely to grow or spread)	Static Vascular Malformations (likely to stay the same)
Hemangiomas	Simple or combined
Kaposiform hemangioendothelioma	Arterial
Tufted angioma	Venous
Kaposi's sarcoma	Capillary
Angiosarcoma	Lymphatic

Figure 6 Classification of vascular anomalies. Adapted from: Chang, MW. Updated Classification of Hemangiomas and Other Vascular Anomalies (adapted from ISSVA classification).

her development. The most commonly seen proliferative vascular anomalies are:

- Hemangiomas are the most frequently seen vascular anomaly. They are not very evident at birth, grow for several months, then stabilize and involute ("diminish") on their own.

- **Kaposiform hemangioendotheliomas** and **tufted angiomas** differ from hemangiomas in appearance and clinical presentation. Both of these lesions may be associated with abnormalities in blood counts and clotting factors. A kaposiform hemangioendothelioma (KHE) is often a boggy, usually purplish, sometimes leathery mass, and may develop **lymphedema**. A tufted angioma (TA) may appear as a leathery-textured purple red patch on the surface of the skin. Platelets and other factors may be "consumed" within these lesions in a process termed **Kasabach–Merritt phenomenon**. Biopsy can confirm the diagnosis. These vascular anomalies are discussed in more detail in the following questions.

Kaposiform hemangioendothelioma (KHE)

Boggy vascular lesion often associated with Kasabach-Merritt phenomenon.

Tufted angiomas

Vascular lesion localized to the skin and underlying tissues; may feel "leathery" and be associated with Kasabach-Merritt phenomenon.

Lymphedema

Swelling from blocked lymphatic vessels or lymph node problems.

Kasabach-Merritt phenomenon

Term for when a vascular tumor consumes blood products including platelets and clotting factors.

Johanna says:

I knew very little, in fact nothing, about this illness when my daughter was diagnosed with it. I was just scared and astounded by what I saw on my angel's head. I later learned, through my daughter's specialist and my own research, that this big red and brown tumor–looking mass on her head was improperly developed blood vessels that grow to become this tumor on the skin. As the days went by, we learned that this tumor also causes low platelet count and is very dangerous. It is an illness that is very complex and needs to be treated immediately.

The Basics

The most frequently seen proliferative type of vascular anomaly is a "typical" hemangioma of infancy. Although adults are often told they have hemangiomas in the liver, spleen, spine, or other locations, strictly speaking these are vascular malformations. Hemangiomas of infancy are rather common and are seen in approximately 7–13% of newborns. Typical hemangiomas are either not evident or appear at birth as a flat pink or white area or a red dot. They increase in size and bulkiness over several months, then gradually involute. The end result after involution depends on the location and other factors related to the type of hemangioma. Further evaluation or treatment of hemangiomas of infancy depends on the location and/or related complications or impending complications.

A subset of patients with hemangiomas undergo extensive evaluation for associated clinical findings, such as those at risk for **PHACES association**. PHACES is an acronym for the following abnormalities:

> **Posterior fossa** structural brain anomalies
> **H**emangiomas in a "segmental" distribution
> **A**rterial anomalies
> **C**ardiac anomalies
> **E**ye abnormalities
> **S**ternal or other midline anomalies and/or spinal axis involvement

For more about PHACES, see Question 69.

Other types of infantile hemangiomas, called **RICH** (**r**apidly **i**nvoluting **c**ongenital **h**emangiomas) and **NICH** (**n**oninvoluting **c**ongenital **h**emangiomas), undergo a different clinical course. These lesions are all benign and are discussed further in subsequent questions.

PHACES association

Acronym that refers to an association of symptoms that occur in common patterns involving anomalies of the posterior fossa or brain, hemangiomas in a "segmental" distribution, arterial anomalies, cardiac anomalies, eye abnormalities, and sternal or other midline abnormalities.

Posterior fossa

Area at base of the skull containing brain stem and cerebellum.

RICH

Subtype of hemangioma that grows in utero and is large at birth, then gradually improves over time; may have high blood flow.

NICH

Noninvoluting congenital hemangioma.

Vascular malformations are congenital abnormalities of the blood vessel development. They are not malignant. They can be isolated, involving one vessel type (capillary, venous, arterial, lymphatic), or combined type (such as venolymphatic malformation, **arteriovenous malformation, capillary malformation**). While some vascular anomalies are superficial such as a capillary malformation (or a "port wine stain") involving the skin only, other vascular anomalies are not apparent unless visualized with a radiologic study, often via magnetic resonance imaging (MRI).

Some vascular anomalies may cause symptoms before birth (e.g., high-flow hemangiomas in the liver, high-flow RICH-type hemangiomas, vein of Galen anomalies in the brain, large arteriovenous malformations). Prenatal **ultrasound** may also identify related structural anomalies that cause no symptoms such as cysts of **lymphatic malformations**, vascular malformation-associated skeletal hypertrophy, extra or missing digits, leg asymmetries, and other findings.

Another lesion often mislabeled as a hemangioma is a pyogenic granuloma, which is a small nodule, often on the face, which bleeds. This typically appears in an older child and can be removed by a simple outpatient surgical procedure.

While vascular anomalies can affect a person's appearance, they generally are not simply cosmetic problems. Proper evaluation is crucial to determine the clinical significance and extent of a vascular anomaly. There are several **syndromes** associated with vascular malformations that are further described in Question 26.

Arteriovenous malformation

Arteriovenous malformations occur when arteries are directly connected to veins without the normal capillary bed between them to slow down the velocity of blood flow.

Capillary malformation

Dilation of a cluster of small blood vessels (capillaries), which results in a visible reddish or purplish coloring of the skin; also called a port wine stain, it is present at birth.

Ultrasound

Medical imaging test used to visualize soft tissue by using sound waves.

Lymphatic malformation (LM)

Abnormal growth of channels and vessels that transport clear, protein-rich lymphatic fluid.

Syndrome

Grouping of physical findings and symptoms occurring together distinguishing a specific disorder, disease.

The Basics

7. How do vascular anomalies affect a person's circulatory system?

Patients with vascular anomalies have differences in blood and/or lymphatic vessels. Based on the location(s) and complications (which are either already present or are anticipated to arise), there may be visible changes to a person's appearance (which may cause functional impairment) and/or abnormalities of the functions of these vessels. Arteriovenous malformations, **hepatic** hemangiomas with **shunting**, or high-flow hemangiomas may cause a "high-flow state" manifesting as the heart having to work harder. A cardiologist will help determine if medications are required to help the heart handle the increased flow. Patients with PHACES association may have abnormally shaped arteries in the brain. Patients with certain types of venous anomalies may have poorly developed deep vessels in the legs. In general, however, the body compensates by creating alternate (collateral) flow patterns so blood flows to where it must. The vessels in patients with these types of abnormalities must be monitored regularly with different tests. Most patients with vascular anomalies, though, have few cardiovascular effects.

Hepatic

Pertaining to the liver.

Shunting

Occurs when blood flows directly from arteries to veins without intervening capillaries.

8. What causes vascular anomalies?

The majority of vascular anomalies appear to be sporadic (that is, there is no specific known cause). Rarely, multiple family members have had hemangiomas; when this occurs, researchers have been able to gain insight into potential genetic predispositions to hemangiomas and other vascular lesions. In recent years, a number of genetic mutations have been identified in patients and family members with vascular anomalies, thus enabling specialists to offer genetic counseling to these families. Often the mutation is found in the patient and one parent who may not have clinical evidence of the anomaly.

Table 1   Genetic Mutations in Vascular Anomalies

Disorder	Gene	Finding
Capillary malformation—arteriovenous malformation (CM-AVM)	RASA-1	Arteriovenous malformation (AVM) plus small pink-red areas on many areas of the skin (capillary malformation)
Familial lymphedema: Milroy's—type 1	VEGF-Flt-4	Congenital lymphedema, presents with swelling of one or both feet or legs
Meige's—type 2	FOX-C2	Lymphedema presenting at or after puberty (also called lymphedema praecox or lymphedema tarda)
Lymphedema dyschiasias	FOX-C2	Distichiasis (extra eyelashes) and lymphedema of extremities, may have other congenital developmental anomalies
Hereditary hemorrhagic telangiectasia (HHT)	Endoglin	Pulmonary AVMs
	ALK-1	Liver AVMS more common
	MADH-4	Juvenile polyposis
Familial mucocutaneous venous malformaitons	Tie-2	Venous malformations in mucosal areas (for example, the mouth) and skin

Familial glomovenous malformation:
  Paraganglioma
  Glomovenous malformation
	Glomulin	Distinct type of blue-purple compressible plaque-like vascular malformation of the skin, usually multifocal, characterized by the presence of glomus cells; may be painful

Familial cerebral cavernous malformation (CCM):
  CCM-1
  CCM-2
  CCM-3
	
	KRIT
	Malcaverin
	PDCD10
		Collections of abnormally formed thin-walled blood vessels in the brain, that are prone to bleed; can be multifocal

Table 1 lists genetic mutations that have been identified thus far, and Question 32 discusses this topic in further detail.

Since the surfaces of "typical" hemangioma cells contain similar proteins to placental cells, an intriguing

Fetus
Development after embryo stage and prior to birth.

hypothesis suggests that (some) hemangiomas may be due to placenta cells dislodging and settling in the **fetus**. This theory has not been proven.

9. How common are vascular anomalies?

Approximately one in ten children are born with a hemangioma.

Approximately one in ten children are born with a hemangioma. Of these children, about half will require medical intervention of some type. Because hemangiomas are not typically present at birth, they are not listed on birth registries. Most hemangiomas are harmless and require observation at most. Early referral to specialists for potentially at-risk patients can help expedite the appropriate evaluation and management, and in some cases can prevent undue complications such as airway and vision problems. At the very least, early referral can provide families with reassurance about the diagnosis. Vascular malformations may not be evident at birth; for example, certain types of lymphedema or malformations may become evident in the adolescent years.

Many syndromes occur in conjunction with vascular anomalies. These are discussed in detail throughout this book.

10. What is the history of the field of vascular anomalies?

Vascular anomalies are not new. Throughout history, there have been references to vascular anomalies, yet the study of these disorders has not traditionally been emphasized in medical training. In recent years, however, research in the mechanisms of blood vessel growth and development has led to therapies to inhibit unwanted vessel growth (as seen in cancers and other disorders) as well as to stimulate new vessel growth (for example in areas of damaged tissue such as the cardiac muscle after a heart attack). Researchers have also discovered new insights into the genetic components of vascular and lymphatic development.

The International Society for the Study of Vascular Anomalies (www.issva.org) was founded in 1992 by a core group of physicians of multiple specialties who shared an interest and expertise in vascular anomalies. This group, with an increasing membership, has contributed greatly to the nomenclature and both basic and clinical research in vascular anomalies, and it has served as a catalyst for other practitioners and researchers. Other medical subspecialty societies are incorporating vascular anomalies in the roster of symposia and workshops at national and international professional meetings. Publications in interdisciplinary, peer-reviewed journals are increasing in frequency.

11. How do I find a qualified doctor to diagnose and evaluate a vascular anomaly?

Many patients with vascular anomalies are initially misdiagnosed. In fact, most adult patients who have been told they have a hemangioma actually have a vascular malformation.

Various patient support organizations provide referral information for consumers and prospective patients about vascular anomalies centers and physician specialists. Many of these support organizations provide networking opportunities for families to contact other patients and/or families and were founded by patients and parents of patients. Through a patient support organization, you will be able to find physician specialists who have very focused expertise in a particular type of vascular or lymphatic anomaly. See the Appendix for listings.

12. How does working with a multidisciplinary team of specialists help in the diagnosis of vascular anomalies?

Vascular anomalies are often medically complex, requiring input and treatment by a number of specialists. A multidisciplinary team approach will allow your care to be coordinated among doctors of many specialties. Patients with vascular anomalies often have a number of medical issues that are interrelated. Because members of your treatment team have different areas of expertise, they are able to approach your care comprehensively. They communicate regularly with the other members of the team as well as the primary care provider. Comprehensive treatment by providers who are familiar with vascular anomalies can also be more cost effective, and some insurance companies are recognizing this.

In some institutions, the multidisciplinary team sees patients together in one location. In other medical centers, appointments are made with various specialists sequentially, and the physicians discuss the patients in a "virtual" conference in which they are not all in the same room at the same time. In many centers, patients are also discussed at a group meeting in the absence of the patient, and radiologic tests, photographs, and pathology studies are reviewed by the team, who subsequently recommends a course of treatment. Generally, one physician on the team will be primarily responsible for communicating with the family and following up with the patient. In some hospitals, the dermatologist may be the primary physician; in others, the surgeon or other medical specialist may be.

13. What doctors and specialists will need to be involved?

Patients who have access to a multidisciplinary vascular anomalies program will benefit from early referrals to appropriate experienced subspecialists who work together to coordinate evaluation, treatment, and management.

Depending on a person's individual case, specialists from **interventional radiology**, **cardiology**, plastic surgery, **hematology**, surgery, dermatology, otolaryngology, ophthalmology, orthopedics, **physiatry**, radiology, and other specialty areas may be involved.

Your treatment team may also include nonphysician professionals such as a social worker, a psychologist, a nurse practitioner, or a physician's assistant. See Table 2 for a listing of specialists and their roles.

14. How do I know if the physician performing my treatment procedure is properly qualified?

Through a vascular anomalies center patients benefit from being able to consult with an experienced interdisciplinary team that works together to formulate the best treatment plan for each patient. This collaborative approach provides a system of checks and balances wherein multiple professionals strategize about the best individualized approach. Patients and families may choose to ask the treating physician how long he or she has been specializing in the field and how many patients with vascular anomalies he or she sees. Patients may also ask how often a physician performs a particular procedure.

Interventional radiology

Specialized branch of radiology that studies and treats disorders of the blood vessels by using catheterization.

Cardiology

Branch of medicine dealing with disorders of the heart.

Hematology

Study of the blood and blood diseases.

Physiatry

Area of medicine specializing in physical medicine or rehabilitation.

The Basics

Table 2 Composition of Vascular Anomalies Team

Type of Physician or Health Professional	Role
Radiologist	
General/pediatric	Recommends and interprets results of radiologic studies
Interventional radiologist	Performs venograms and angiograms; can administer treatments within the affected blood vessels
Surgeon	
Plastic surgeon	Performs biopsies, debulking/resection of lesions +/− laser therapy
Otolaryngologist (ear, nose, throat [ENT])	As above, plus visualization of the airway, laser/surgery of airway and tracheostomy placement if needed
General surgeon	Biopsy, debulking, +/− resection of lesions, mediport/broviac placement
Oculoplastic surgeon	Performs resection of lesions affecting the eye area
Orthopedic	Monitors bone growth; performs surgeries as needed to correct limb length discrepancies, hand and foot problems
Dermatologist	
General/pediatric	Diagnostic and therapeutic recommendations, skin biopsies, some intralesional therapies
Laser	Laser therapy for superficial vascular lesions
Medical therapist	
Hematologist/oncologist	Prescribes and monitors medical therapy, including chemotherapy, monitoring blood counts, treating coagulation defects (bleeding or clotting) associated with vascular anomalies
Neurologist	Assesses and monitors neurodevelopment, possible treatment-related toxicity
Ophthalmologist	Evaluates and monitors eye function
Geneticist	When possible, determines genetic basis of disorder, establishes family pedigree and sends blood samples for genetic mutation studies
Physiatrist	Assesses motor and sensory function; recommends orthotics and/or physical therapy regimen

Table 2   Composition of Vascular Anomalies Team (Continued)

Type of Physician	Role
Physical therapist	Works with patient regularly for physical therapy, occupational therapy, lymphatic massage therapy
Psychologist	Works with patient and family focusing on adjustment issues related to the treatment and disorders
Social worker	Helps family and patient cope with medical, psychosocial, financial and practical issues
Patient Advocate	Patient/family support, networking with similar cases
Nurse Practitioner or Physician's Assistant	Works with medical team to help facilitate coordinated care

Some patients find reassurance by asking for referral suggestions from a diagnosing physician or through various patient support organizations, which list individual physicians and treatment centers that specialize in these disorders. Many of the physicians have published peer-reviewed journals in this field and teach at their institutions as well as nationally and internationally. They also participate in patient advocacy meetings and lectures/consultations organized by patient support groups. The Appendix lists the major vascular anomalies organizations and services/resources they offer.

15. Should we get a second opinion?

It is your right to obtain further medical opinions. These are best provided by physicians familiar with vascular malformations. Your physician or one of the patient advocacy sites can provide you with names of experts close to where you live. If you are seeking a second opinion, it will be important to bring all pertinent consultant notes, laboratory studies, radiology reports as well as copies of the radiologic studies (often available on a CD), and pathology slides (if relevant). Jot down your specific questions in advance to make the best use of your time.

Do not be surprised if different physicians recommend divergent interventions. There are many gray areas, and physicians will gravitate toward their expertise and experience.

Jessica says:

When our son was born with a large RICH on his buttocks, the pediatric surgeon at the hospital didn't know what it was or what to do about it. He told us, "They are going to tell you that is a hemangioma, but they will be wrong." As it turned out, it was a hemangioma, and thankfully we were able to find doctors who knew what to do about it. If time is available, get a second opinion.

> *Do not be surprised if different physicians recommend divergent interventions. There are many gray areas, and physicians will gravitate toward their expertise and experience.*

16. What are some of the key tests used to identify, diagnose, and classify vascular anomalies?

Experienced vascular anomalies specialists can make the correct diagnosis based on the history, clinical presentation, and appearance of the vascular anomaly. Testing may include blood tests, ultrasound, x-ray, MRI, **lymphoscintigram**, eye examination by an ophthalmologist, bronchoscopy, endoscopy, etc., depending on the location or characteristics of the vascular anomaly. The most frequently ordered diagnostic tests are listed in the Table 3. Typically, photographs will be taken at each visit to document the changes (including response to treatment, if pertinent) in the vascular anomaly over time.

Lymphoscintigram

Test using a radioactive tracer injected into the feet and visualized over several time points to assess if there is an abnormality of lymphatic drainage.

Table 3   Common Diagnostic Radiologic Tests

Radiologic Test	Purpose	Comment
Ultrasound	Can detect flow characteristics, mass, blood clot	Painless No sedation required
MRI (+/− gadolinium [contrast])	Evaluates extent ("tip of the iceberg") and characteristics of vascular lesion and other structural anomalies	Long study Sedation required* Provides in-depth information
MR angiogram (MRA)	Evaluates arteries	Sedation required*
MR venogram (MRV)	Evaluates venous flow	Sedation required*
Computed tomography (CT scan) (+/− contrast)	Evaluates soft tissue, bones	Radiation Contrast material may cause allergic reaction
Angiogram	Real time study of arteries via catheter directly inserted into arteries of interest +/− embolization therapy during angiogram	Requires anesthesia Contrast dye, radiation, complications
Venogram	Real time study of veins of interest via catheter directly inserted into arteries of interest +/− sclerotherapy therapy during angiogram	Requires anesthesia Contrast dye, radiation, complications
Lymphoscintigram	Radioactive albumin injected into foot or hands, then tracked over time to assess lymphatic drainage time and path	Radioactive, limited availability of study, cooperative patient required
DEXA scan (dual-energy x-ray absorptiometry)	Measurement of the amount of low-dose x-rays absorbed to determine bone density	Limited pediatric data (improving)

*For infant > several weeks old until mature enough to remain still for minutes at a time.

The Basics

Sometimes the diagnosis is not clear. A biopsy may be required if there is any question of the diagnosis and **histologic** confirmation is required.

17. When is an ultrasound helpful?

Ultrasound is a simple noninvasive, nonpainful test that does not require sedation. In addition to the routine screening prenatal ultrasounds, ultrasounds may detect vascular anomalies (hepatic, lymphatic, arterial) or structural abnormalities associated with vascular anomalies (e.g., posterior fossa abnormalities associated with PHACES association, limb **hypertrophy** syndromes).

Newborn infants with vascular staining, swelling, excess hair growth, sinus tracts, or other midline findings of the lower back benefit from an ultrasound of the lower spine to rule out the presence of hidden spinal anomalies. The timing of these studies is important; after a few months of age, the resolution of the study is limited as the spinal bones ossify (become calcified), in which case an MRI may be required. MRI confirmation of a suspected anomaly of the spinal cord is also warranted.

Ultrasound evaluation with Doppler flow studies is used for suspected hemangiomas of the liver. Routine ultrasound of cutaneous (skin) vascular lesions is not often diagnostic. In fact, other than documenting blood flow, they may lead to false reassurance. If there is any question as to the diagnosis, MRI and/or biopsy should be considered.

Doppler ultrasound is also used when **deep venous thrombosis** is suspected. Some centers also use Doppler and ultrasound to assess flow characteristics of vascular anomalies in the arms and legs (extremities).

Histology

Assessment of the cell organization and structure, as seen under the microscope.

Hypertrophy

Enlarged body part.

Deep venous thrombosis

Blood clot in deep venous system.

18. What is an MRI?

MRI stands for **magnetic resonance imaging**. This technology uses a magnetic field and radio waves to create detailed, high-resolution images of organs and structures within the body. When a person lies in an MRI machine, a magnetic field causes atoms within the body to align in a particular way. Radio waves are then applied to the body, or a part of the body, which cause the aligned particles to transmit a signal. A scanner then receives these signals and interprets them to produce three-dimensional images.

MRI scans are useful because they are noninvasive, do not expose patients to radiation, and provide useful information that other imaging tests cannot. In most cases, an MRI scan is performed with a contrast medium (gadolinium), to better visualize blood vessels and tissues. A radiologist reviews these images and can interpret the findings to delineate the extent and flow characteristics of disorders, including vascular anomalies.

Young children require anesthesia/sedation to ensure they do not move during the study. Infants a few weeks old may benefit from a "feed and wrap" protocol whereby they are fed immediately before the study. They are then swaddled to encourage them to fall asleep naturally during the study, thus preventing the need for anesthesia.

19. How is a computed tomography (CT) scan used?

A CT, or CAT, scan is a diagnostic imaging technique by which multiple x-rays are taken from different angles and then combined by a computer to create very

Magnetic resonance imaging

Special type of MR study focusing on the arterial structure.

The Basics

detailed cross-sectional images of internal structures of the body. In some cases contrast dye may be used to make the pictures clearer or to provide greater detail. As with any x-ray, patients are exposed to radiation during the procedure; however, most centers minimize the radiation dosing in small children.

CT scans may be used for patients with vascular anomalies in order to study bony changes better that are not well visualized with an MRI.

PART TWO

Vascular Malformations

What is a vascular malformation?

What are some of the syndromes
related to vascular malformations?

What are some medications used to treat
patients with vascular malformations?

More . . .

20. What is a vascular malformation?

Vascular malformations can affect veins, arteries, capillaries, and even lymphatic vessels. Vascular malformations are generally present prior to birth and grow in parallel with the overall growth of the patient. They are benign, or noncancerous, lesions. Even if they are present at birth, they may not become obvious until later, depending on the type and location of the malformation.

Vascular malformations affect males and females in equal frequency and can be located in any part of the body including the trunk, extremities, face, brain, or internal organs. They can affect one or several parts of the vascular system (e.g., they may affect the capillaries and veins, but not the arteries or lymphatic vessels) and are most precisely described based on the involved vessels. Clearly those affecting the skin are evident at birth.

Vascular anomalies are diagnosed through a variety of techniques. Sometimes vascular anomalies are obvious on the surface of the skin. With a thorough history and physical examination, a physician may be able to make the correct diagnosis by looking and touching the vascular anomaly. Sometimes, if the diagnosis is not obvious or typical, further testing is required, including blood tests, radiologic studies (e.g., ultrasound, x-rays, MRI). Sometimes a biopsy, which is a procedure to remove part of the lesion for diagnostic purposes, is required. In that case, a pathologist will look at the lesion under the microscope to examine the cells making up the vascular lesion and determine the diagnosis.

Figures 7 and 8 provide images of patients with different vascular malformations.

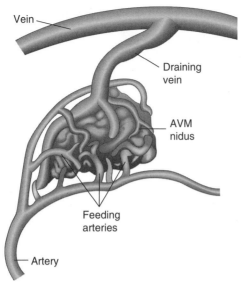

Figure 7   An arteriovenous malformation (AVM).

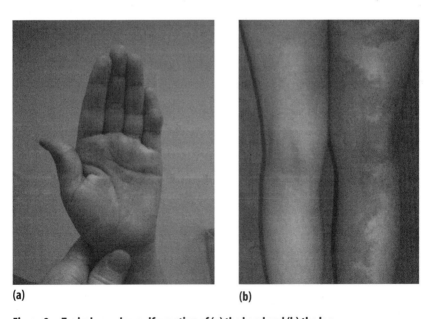

(a)   (b)

Figure 8   Typical vascular malformation of (a) the hand and (b) the leg.

21. What is the typical natural history of a vascular malformation?

The major difference between hemangiomas and vascular malformations is that the latter do not involute and are present throughout the patient's lifetime. However, similar to hemangiomas, where they are located in the body and their clinical features determine how they are medically evaluated and managed.

For example, a **capillary malformation** (also called a port wine stain) presenting on the arm or abdomen may not cause concern, but one that covers the upper half or the entire face warrants evaluation for Sturge-Weber syndrome. Likewise, the presence of a large lymphatic malformation of the neck would require evaluation to monitor for airway compromise. High-flow vascular malformations such as arteriovenous malformations may present acutely with heart failure from arterial shunting and/or hydrocephalus due to blockage of cerebrospinal fluid drainage, as is the case with vein of Galen malformations in the brain.

The vast majority of vascular malformations are not *associated with cancer.*

22. Are vascular malformations cancerous?

While patients with rare vascular malformation syndromes (such as Maffucci syndrome or PTEN-associated vascular malformations) may be predisposed to malignancies in adulthood, the vast majority of vascular malformations are *not* associated with cancer.

23. What are PTEN-associated vascular malformations?

PTEN stands for *phosphatase and tensin homolog protein,* encoded by the PTEN gene. PTEN is a tumor suppressor gene. In the normal state, PTEN prevents rapid cell growth. When mutated, this function of

PTEN behaves abnormally, making patients with the PTEN mutation susceptible to cancers. Some patients with vascular anomalies have the PTEN mutation, such as those with Cowden syndrome and Bannayan-Riley-Ruvalcaba syndrome, and some patients with proteus syndrome. Some patients with vascular malformations may have the **PTEN hamartoma tumor syndrome (PHTS)**, which represents a spectrum of disorders.

These syndromes are suspected if there are lipomas (benign fatty tumors), thyroid disorders, characteristic skin lesions, macrocephaly (large head), penile **lentigines** (freckles on the penis), or other associated findings. The only way to confirm the syndromes is to have a blood sample sent for PTEN mutational analysis; although there are several possible mutations, only the most common mutations can be tested. If an individual tests positive for this mutation, other family members will be tested, and early screening for thyroid, breast, brain, gynecologic, and other cancers will be initiated for those with the PTEN mutation.

Cowden syndrome is a rare disorder characterized by multiple noncancerous (benign) growths called hamartomas and an increased risk of developing certain cancers. Vascular malformations may be lymphatic, venous, or other. The skin growths, which are usually small, usually appear in the 20s, may look like warts or skin tags, and can be found on the skin and the mucous membranes (mouth, cheeks, gums, nasal passages).

Malignancies seen in patients with Cowden syndrome are usually breast, thyroid, or endometrium (lining of the uterus). Benign tumors are also seen in patients with Cowden syndrome—thyroid nodules, breast masses,

PTEN hamartoma tumor syndrome (PHTS)

Cluster of clinical findings (see Cowden syndrome and Bannayan-Riley-Ruvalcaba syndrome) associated with PTEN mutation.

Lentigines

Freckles.

Cowden syndrome

Disorder characterized by macrocephaly, hamartomas, skin tag-appearing lesions, thyroid nodules, lipomas (benign fatty lumps) and/or cancers, and vascular malformations.

and a noncancerous brain tumor called Lhermitte-Duclos disease (LDD), also referred to as dysplastic gangliocytoma of the cerebellum). Patients with Cowden syndrome may have a large head and cognitive delays. The diagnosis is often made in adolescence or early adulthood.

Often the suspicion of Cowden syndrome begins with a family history of thyroid nodules, lipomas (benign fatty lumps), and/or cancers, as previously noted. If the family history and clinical spectrum (macrocephaly, hamartomas, skin tag-appearing lesions) are present, the patient and family should be referred to a genetics specialist for further discussion and blood testing for the presence of the PTEN mutation. Since not all the mutations are available for testing, more sophisticated tests may be required if the initial test is negative and the patient/family fulfills the criteria for the disorder. Upon the suspicion or diagnosis of Cowden syndrome, individuals should be placed in a cancer surveillance program to facilitate early detection and prompt referral for further evaluation and treatment.

Bannayan-Riley-Ruvalcaba syndrome is characterized by macrocephaly (enlarged head), noncancerous fatty masses (lipomas), vascular malformations, intestinal polyps, thyroid disorders, pectus excavatum (caved-in appearing breast bone), hyperextensible joints, proximal muscle abnormalities, and predisposition to breast and thyroid cancers. Male patients have freckles on the penis. Bannayan-Riley-Ruvalcaba syndrome is also associated with mutations of the PTEN gene, thus the same guidelines hold true for patients suspected of having this disorder, as well as their family members. Bannayan-Riley-Ruvalcaba syndrome is often diagnosed in childhood.

Bannayan-Riley-Ruvalcaba syndrome

Macrocephaly (enlarged head), noncancerous fatty masses (lipomas), vascular malformations, intestinal polyps, thyroid disorders, pectus excavatum (caved-in appearing breast bone), hyperextensible joints, proximal muscle abnormalities, and predisposition to breast and thyroid cancers. Male patients have freckles on the penis.

Cowden syndrome and Bannayan-Riley-Ruvalcaba syndrome are inherited in an **autosomal dominant** fashion; thus, having only one copy of this abnormal gene is sufficient to manifest the disorder. Genetic testing can determine if other family members are affected or if this is a spontaneous mutation occurring only in the patient.

24. Are vascular malformations painful?

Day-to-day, vascular malformations are not usually painful. Patients may experience a sense of fullness, due to swelling, after walking or standing for prolonged periods. Use of **compression stockings** or wraps, or keeping the extremity elevated may decrease the discomfort. Phleboliths are calcifications of the remains of localized clots and only appear in a delayed fashion after the acute event. They are sometimes painful and can be relieved with oral ibuprofen-containing medications such as Advil or Motrin.

Development of a deep venous thrombosis is often associated with calf pain (or pain elsewhere depending on the location of the affected vessel). A Doppler study can document the blood clot. Anticoagulation therapy must be started promptly to prevent further clotting and possible dislodgement of the clot, which would travel to the lungs (causing a pulmonary embolism). Pain can also occur if a vascular malformation is located adjacent to a nerve, causing irritation and painful sensations.

In the peripubertal years, patients often experience bouts of discomfort, presumably due to hormonal changes to which the endothelial cells of the vascular malformations are sensitive.

Autosomal dominant

Inheritance of a gene on a non-sex chromosome (i.e. not the X or Y chromosome) from one parent resulting in disease.

Compression stockings

Therapeutic device used to support the venous and lymphatic system of the leg.

Vascular Malformations

25. Is a port wine stain birthmark a vascular malformation?

Yes. A port wine stain is another term for capillary or venular malformations. These lesions are discolored areas on the surface of skin that range in color from pale pink to dark purple and are present at birth. They grow slowly at the rate of a child and do not spread to other areas. Over time they may become darker and thicker, especially if untreated.

Laser therapy is an effective treatment for port wine stains, but often a series of treatments is needed to produce a significant change. Lifelong maintenance treatments are usually required to maintain the lightened effect.

Depending on where port wine stains are located on the body, they may be a sign of Sturge-Weber syndrome or Klippel-Trenaunay syndrome, indicating that further neurologic and/or ophthalmologic evaluation is necessary.

26. What are some of the syndromes related to vascular malformations?

In addition to the rare PTEN-associated vascular anomaly-hamartoma syndrome, there are more common vascular anomaly syndromes as listed in the Table 4.

Sturge-Weber Syndrome

Sturge-Weber syndrome (SWS) is suspected when an infant is born with a facial capillary malformation. This malformation appears as a flat pink/red stain, and it can involve one or both sides of the face. Seizures, **focal** neurologic deficits (weakness, numbness, hemi-blindness) **contralateral** to the facial lesion, developmental delay,

Sturge-Weber syndrome (SWS)

Medical condition with facial capillary malformation, often associated with seizures and glaucoma.

Focal

Occurring in one location.

Contralateral

Occurring on the opposite side.

Table 4   Vascular Malformation Syndromes

Syndrome	Features
Klippel-Trenaunay syndrome (extremities +/− trunk)	Capillary malformation on surface of skin +/− lymphatic blebs (small cysts filled with lymphatic fluid)
	Venous +/− lymphatic malformation—may have varicose (dilated) veins, +/− poorly developed deep venous system
	Asymmetry of extremities (usually affected extremity is larger in girth, possible limb length discrepancy), +/− other abnormalities of digits/toes
Gorham syndrome ("disappearing bone disease")	Replacement of normal bone by abnormal lymphatic growth which destroys the bone
Maffucci syndrome (Ollier disease)	Multifocal enchondromas (enlargement of cartilage), vascular malformations, other benign vascular masses presenting as lumps, limb abnormalities, may predispose to malignancy
Proteus syndrome	Focal limb and soft tissue overgrowth, unusual thickening of soles of feet, nevi (moles), vascular malformations
Macrocephaly (capillary malformation syndrome)	Macrocephaly (large head circumference) and capillary malformations with ≥ 2 of the following: limb asymmetry, developmental delay, facial midline capillary malformation, congenital hypotonia (poor tone), syndactyly/polydactyly, prominent forehead, joint hypermobility/hyperelastic skin, and/or hydrocephalus
Hereditary hemorrhagic telangiectasia (Osler-Weber-Rendu syndrome)	Multifocal arteriovenous malformations (telangiectasias) on skin, mucous membranes (e.g., nasal passages) +/− internal organs—gastrointestinal tract, brain, lungs, liver; often causes bleeding
Sturge-Weber syndrome	Facial capillary malformation, glaucoma, seizures
Blue rubber bleb nevus syndrome	Multiple small venous malformations, including throughout gastrointestinal tract +/− other organs—may cause bleeding

and glaucoma and may be associated with Sturge-Weber syndrome. Brain imaging has a typical pattern with areas of blood vessel proliferation (**leptomeningeal** angiomatosis), brain atrophy and calcification. Sturge-Weber syndrome occurs equally in males and females. While a predisposing genetic mutation has not yet been identified, investigators are studying potential candidate genes which may be associated with this disorder. Some patients also have vascular staining on other parts of the body; however this is not a criterion for Sturge-Weber syndrome.

Another name for Sturge-Weber syndrome is *encephalotrigem-inal angiomatosis,* as the full expression of the disorder includes the facial capillary malformation following the **trigeminal nerve** distribution, in addition to increased vascular growth in the leptomeningeal area of the brain. Seizures, glaucoma, and developmental delay, as well as various comorbidities such as attention deficit hyperactivity disorder (ADHD), depression, and hormonal abnormalities may be associated with Sturge-Weber syndrome. Glaucoma, the presence of increased intraocular pressure, if untreated can damage the optic nerve and cause blindness. Glaucoma can cause *buphthalmos,* enlargement of the affected corneas and eyeball.

Glaucoma may occur at any time and is often asymptomatic; therefore, patients must be monitored closely by an experienced ophthalmologist or glaucoma specialist, more frequently during infancy and early childhood, then minimally one to two times per year. Specifically, the ophthalmologist will check the intraocular pressure, which is elevated in glaucoma.

Researchers have found that MRI or MRA (**magnetic resonance angiogram**) brain imaging as well as a

Leptomeningeal

Referring to the leptomeninges, one of the layers covering the brain.

Trigeminal nerve

Fifth cranial nerve with three major branches, mainly controlling feeling in the face (also controls some movements).

Magnetic resonance angiogram

Special type of MR study focusing on the arterial structure.

technique called quantitative EEG, or qEEG, can reveal important information about possible neurologic involvement. Neurologic symptoms may be acute (seizures) or subtle (onset of developmental delay). It is recommended that children at risk for Sturge-Weber syndrome be evaluated and followed regularly by an experienced neurologist who can discuss emergency measures in the event of a seizure and also the possible medical, educational, and social implications of this disorder. There are many different types of seizures. Medications used to treat seizures are called antiepileptics. Although general neurologists treat patients with seizures, neurologists who specialize in treating patients with seizures are called epileptologists. When medications are not able to control seizures, a patient may be evaluated for a vagal nerve stimulator implant or surgical resection of the seizure focus if indicated.

There are three categories of Sturge-Weber syndrome:

- **Type 1:** This type involves the face, brain, and eyes. These patients are prone to seizures, especially if both sides of the face are affected by the capillary malformation. The eye involvement may initially manifest as "red eye," or extra capillaries on the surface of the sclera (white portion of the eyeball). Patients with all three anatomic areas of involvement are at highest risk for neurologic symptoms, including developmental delay.
- **Type 2:** This type involves a facial vascular staining with a normal brain and possible glaucoma.
- **Type 3:** In these patients, the *forme fruste* (incomplete, unusual) type of Sturge-Weber syndrome, there is brain involvement without cutaneous (skin) findings or glaucoma.

Not every child with a facial capillary malformation has Sturge-Weber syndrome. As noted, the risk increases when both sides of the face are involved. The National Institutes of Health and The Sturge-Weber Foundation provide helpful medical information and resources at their Web sites:

- www.ninds.nih.gov (Search for "Sturge-Weber.")
- www.sturgeweber.kennedykrieger.org
- www.sturge-weber.org

The last Web site, for The Sturge-Weber Foundation (www.sturge-weber.org), has a host of resources for patients, including educational printed and audio-visual materials in English and multilingual translations, log books for medical visits and treatments, emergency room guides, online networking blogs, and suggestions for working with insurance companies.

Some researchers are conducting radiologic studies as well as testing if different medications and diet can prevent or modify symptoms such as seizures in patients with Sturge-Weber syndrome. There are other Sturge-Weber Foundation–funded researchers working on developing a mouse model and investigating immune suppression and hormone abnormalities. The Sturge-Weber Foundation Web site lists these centers as well as research projects they have recently funded.

Flashlamp pulsed dye laser treatments

Laser treatment that improves red color of superficial vascular lesions; may prevent outward growth of early hemangiomas.

Should your child be suspected of having Sturge-Weber syndrome, he or she will be referred to an ophthalmologist for regular visits, a neurologist to follow neurodevelopment and to discuss the possibility of seizures and their management, and a laser specialist, who can help lighten or eradicate the capillary malformation with **flashlamp pulsed dye laser treatments**.

Management will then be tailored around the clinical findings and symptoms, if present. The Sturge-Weber Foundation has designated "Sturge-Weber Centers of Excellence," and these institutions have teams of doctors and support staff who have expertise in this disorder.

Klippel-Trenaunay Syndrome

Klippel-Trenaunay syndrome (KTS), a relatively common vascular anomaly syndrome, is named after the two French physicians who first described this disorder in 1900, Maurice Klippel and Paul Trénaunay. This syndrome describes a vascular malformation syndrome with anomalies of the vessels of an extremity (more commonly a lower extremity), hypertrophy of the affected extremity, and red or blue changes of the skin. These malformations may be associated with small **blebs** that ooze. Some patients with Klippel-Trenaunay syndrome do not have a well-developed deep venous system. This is important to determine (usually by MRI), as the vessels close to the skin's surface become dominant. Patients with Klippel-Trenaunay syndrome may also have lymphatic malformations or skeletal abnormalities such as extra digits, fused digits, or large feet or hands. Some patients also have anomalies of the abdominal, pelvic, and cranial vessels. Treatment is generally to relieve symptoms of pain and to prevent bleeding, clotting, and/or infections. Problems that can arise in these patients include limb length and girth discrepancies, blood clots, bleeding, cellulitis, lymphedema, and pain. However, day to day, many patients do very well. The medical team involved with patients having Klippel-Trenaunay syndrome often includes an orthopedist, interventional radiologist, dermatologist, hematologist, surgeon, and physiatrist. Helpful information can be found by searching for

Vascular Malformations

Klippel-Trenaunay syndrome (KTS)

Vascular malformation syndrome associated with superficial vascular staining, hypertrophy of an extremity, and underlying venous and/or lymphatic malformation.

Blebs

A blisterlike small cystic structure; may ooze or bleed.

"Klippel-Trenaunay" on the Web sites of the following organizations:

- The Klippel-Trenaunay Syndrome Support Group
- National Institute of Neurological Disorders and Stroke
- Children's Hospital Boston
- KT Foundation
- The Sturge-Weber Foundation
- MedlinePlus

Proteus Syndrome

Proteus syndrome (PS) or proteus-like syndrome is a congenital, asymmetric, disproportionate, and progressive postnatal overgrowth syndrome affecting bone, connective tissue, fat, and organs. Skin manifestations include characteristic cerebriform (brain-like configuration) changes, usually on the soles of the feet, and "linear epidermal nevus," a brown, thick skin lesion. Hands and/or feet may exhibit **gigantism** (outsized growth). Patients with proteus syndrome have dysregulation of fatty tissue, with areas of fatty overgrowth alternating with fat atrophy; characteristic facial features; and capillary, venous, and/or lymphatic malformations. These individuals are at increased risk for malignancies. Proteus syndrome appears to occur sporadically and is considered a **mosaic condition**, which means individuals have a blend of affected (carrying a mutation) and unaffected cells. A multidisciplinary medical team, including a geneticist and orthopedist, is necessary for the proper monitoring and care of these patients.

Gigantism
Excessive growth.

Mosaic condition
Individuals have a blend of affected (carrying a mutation) and unaffected cells.

Web sites with information about proteus syndrome include:

- Proteus Syndrome Foundation
- National Organization for Rare Disorders

Other Syndromes Related to Vascular Malformations

Macrocephaly-capillary malformation is an association of enlarged head (**macrocephaly**) with reticulated (network/weblike) capillary malformation, often with a midline facial vascular stain. Syndactyly (joined digits) and other abnormalities may be present.

Patients with **blue rubber bleb nevus syndrome** have **multifocal** venous malformations involving the skin, gastrointestinal (GI) tract, and soft tissues. **Anemia** often develops due to chronic bleeding from vascular malformations in the gastrointestinal tract. This symptom may manifest as dark or blood-coated stools, and patients may require blood transfusion to replace blood losses.

Patients with blue rubber bleb nevus syndrome have small protuberant soft dark blue discrete rubbery masses, evident on the skin and mucous membranes in areas such as the mouth and lips. Gastrointestinal lesions can be diagnosed by "capsule endoscopy" or "capsule enteroscopy" by which a tiny wireless camera inside a vitamin-sized capsule is swallowed by the patient or inserted by a gastroenterologist. Photographs of the intestinal tract are taken as the device travels throughout the digestive tract. The images are recorded on a monitor that enables the gastroenterologist to identify any abnormalities, including vascular malformations. Successful removal of problematic lesions by experienced surgeons has been described. Other vascular lesions in these patients may respond to sclerotherapy.

Maffucci syndrome is characterized by multifocal firm asymmetric subcutaneous **enchondromas** and dyschondroplasia; improper formation of bone in cartilage; and venous, lymphatic, or other vascular anomalies, including

---

Vascular Malformations

Macrocephaly
Enlarged head.

Blue rubber bleb nevus syndrome
Condition with raised bluish nodules on the skin and throughout the gastrointestinal tract; may cause bleeding.

Multifocal
Occurring in more than one location.

Anemia
Low red blood cell count, leading to pallor.

Maffucci syndrome
Disorder characterized by multifocal firm asymmetric subcutaneous enchondromas and dyschondroplasia, improper formation of bone in cartilage, and venous, lymphatic, or other vascular anomalies.

Enchondromas
Benign tumor of the cartilage.

hemangioendotheliomas. The affected bones in patients with Maffucci syndrome have distinctive x-ray findings. They may suffer severe deforming orthopedic problems including limb length discrepancies, painful vascular nodules, and an increased incidence of cancers, including malignant transformation of enchondromas to chondrosarcomas, as well as cancers of the brain, breast, and genitourinary tract. Thus, these patients warrant early referral for orthopedic follow-up and close monitoring for early detection of cancer due to the 15–20% incidence of malignancies.

27. How does an angiogram help diagnose vascular malformations?

An angiogram is an imaging procedure that allows doctors to see blood vessels, including arteries and veins, and how blood moves within them (Figure 9).

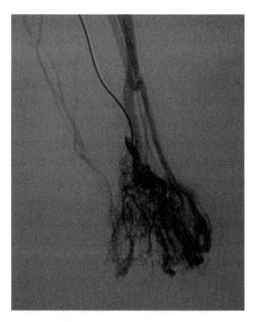

Figure 9   Angiogram of hand and arm AVM.

This procedure is performed in a hospital setting by an interventional radiologist (a physician). During the procedure, the patient is sedated or put under anesthesia. The physician punctures the artery with a needle and a wire is threaded through the needle and into the vessels. Then a catheter (tube) is passed over the wire. A dye (contrast material) is injected into the vessel to allow the doctor to take x-rays of the vessels and their blood flow. This procedure can identify blockages, enlargements, and malformed vessels. Doctors may also be able to treat a problem during an angiogram, such as dissolving a clot by infusing a medication or performing an embolization to close off an unwanted vascular channel through the same catheter.

Angiogram is the general term for this test. If the test studies veins, it is called a **venogram**. If the arteries are studied, the test is called an arteriogram. After the procedure, the physician will review the images showing the malformations with you or your child.

28. What are some treatments for vascular malformations?

Sometimes vascular malformations are removed surgically. This is often the case with small venous malformations or discrete lymphatic malformations. In other cases, embolization or sclerotherapy may be indicated; these therapies are utilized for arteriovenous, venous, and lymphatic malformations. Often management issues are discussed on a case-by-case basis among the involved physicians on the vascular anomalies team. In some cases, no treatment or intervention is required at all. New medical therapies may be available in a research setting.

Venogram
Diagnostic imaging test performed by an interventional radiologist. A catheter is inserted into the vessels of interest, and a contrast dye is injected to directly view blood flow of the venous system.

In some cases, no treatment or intervention for vascular malformations is required at all.

29. How does embolization or sclerotherapy treat a vascular malformation?

Embolization and **sclerotherapy** are procedures that selectively close off blood vessels of a vascular malformation. Usually the treating physician, an interventional radiologist, will identify and map the vessels to be treated during an angiogram or venogram. If indicated, a substance will be injected using the same catheter to block the vessels in question or cause a local clot to shrink the lesion. Agents that are injected include **ethanol**, **bleomycin**, **doxycycline**, n-butyl-2-cyanoacrylate (n-BCA), ethylene-vinyl alcohol copolymer (Onyx), **picibanil**, and others. Sometimes sclerotherapy is performed via direct puncture into the lesion if it is superficially located and easily visualized. Embolization or sclerotherapy can be an effective treatment for vascular lesions in the brain or other parts of the body in the following conditions:

- Venous malformations
- Arteriovenous malformations
- Klippel-Trenaunay syndrome
- Kaposiform hemangioendothelioma
- Conditions in which bleeding needs to be minimized prior to surgical procedures

30. Are there complications that can occur from treatment?

The risks and benefits of any intervention must be weighed. In the case of vascular malformations, the risks of treatment will depend on the affected location and extent of the lesion, age of the patient, any associated symptoms, and many other individual factors. These

Embolization

Procedure by which a solution is injected into abnormal blood vessels or structures to create an obstruction or clot to close off the veins.

Sclerotherapy

Injection of a solution into abnormal blood vessels or structures to create an obstruction or clot to close off the vein.

Ethanol

Alcohol, sometimes used for endovascular treatment of vascular malformations.

Bleomycin

Antibiotic medication that may be injected into certain vascular malformations to make them shrink.

Doxycycline

Antibiotic sometimes used for sclerotherapy of vascular malformations.

Picibanil

Substance used for sclerotherapy of some lymphatic malformations.

considerations will be discussed with you in detail by each of the involved physicians.

Some possible complications from surgery for vascular malformations are (1) the risk of malformation regrowth, (2) the loss or reduction of nerve function in an affected area, (3) the possibility of developing or mobilizing a clot, and (4) scarring. Compartment syndrome is a dangerous increase in pressure within a confined space, especially the calf or forearm. If untreated it can cause severe nerve or muscle damage and is a risk associated with surgery, embolization, and sclerotherapy, depending on the affected area. Procedures or diagnostic tests involving contrast dye may pose a risk to people with certain allergies, such as to iodine or shellfish.

Although these risks may sound frightening, many people with vascular anomalies who are treated by experienced specialists have very good outcomes and results with these, and other, procedures. If you have concerns or questions about specific risks associated with an intervention, it is best to discuss them with your physician(s).

31. What blood tests might be performed for patients with vascular malformations?

Because some patients with vascular malformations may have abnormalities in their blood counts, a CBC (complete blood count) may be performed. The white blood cells, which help fight infection, may be high if the patient has an infection. This may be the case in a patient who has a lymphatic malformation, which may be prone to inflammation and infection. Additionally, in patients with large lymphatic malformations, the lymphocyte count may be low.

The platelet count may be low in patients with venous malformations and localized intravascular coagulation (LIC) due to consumption of these blood products within the abnormal vessels. Other laboratory tests that may be abnormal are the coagulation profile (prothrombin time [PT] and partial thromboplastin time [PTT]), including the fibrinogen level (decreased) and the D-dimers and fibrin degradation products (FDPs), which may be elevated. These levels may alert the physician of a new development, and they may be followed serially to assess response to treatment.

Anticoagulants

Medication or drug that prevents blood clotting.

Hematologist

Doctor specializing in treating diseases of the blood and clotting disorders.

For patients treated with **anticoagulants**, certain blood parameters are monitored. Patients treated with low-molecular-weight heparin may be tested for antifactor Xa levels, and the PT/INR is followed in patients treated with Coumadin. Because of these potential blood test abnormalities, a **hematologist** may be involved in you or your child's care. Table 5 lists and describes these blood tests that help in the diagnosis and treatment of vascular malformations. Your physician will discuss these results with you.

Figure 10 depicts the blood vessel with the red blood cell and platelets (cellular components of the blood), in addition to factors involved with regulated clotting of blood.

The schematic of the coagulation cascade (Figure 11) depicts the main tests (activated PTT, PT, fibrinogen, fibrin degradation products) used for screening coagulation function in certain patients with vascular anomalies.

Table 5   Blood Tests for Patients with Vascular Malformations

Test	What Does the Test Evaluate?	Who is Evaluated?
Complete blood count (CBC)	White cell count, red cell count, platelet count	Patients with venous and arteriovenous malformations (AVMs) Patients with lymphatic malformations (may have infection +/− lymphopenia)
Coagulation profile Fibrinogen Fibrin degradation products D-dimers Thrombophilia evaluation	Clotting profile, assessment for breakdown of products of clotting (which may be seen in "activated" endothelium of certain vascular anomalies), risk for developing blood clots	Patients with venous and arteriovenous malformations (AVMs)
Renal profile	Kidney function	Patients undergoing studies with contrast dye

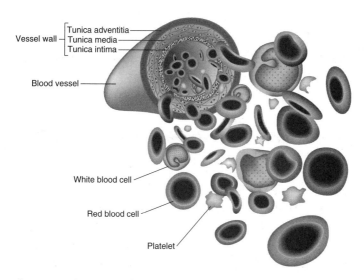

Figure 10   Blood vessel with the cellular components (red cells, white cells, and platelets).

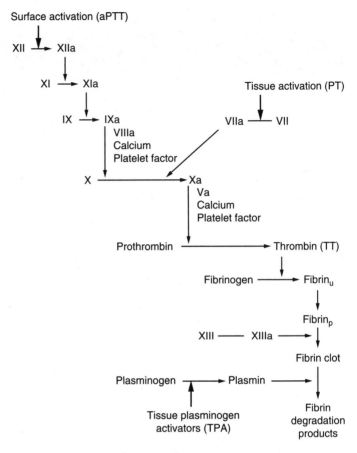

Figure 11   Coagulation cascade showing components modulating human blood clotting.

32. Are vascular malformations inherited, and do genetics play a role?

Sometimes vascular malformations are inherited—that is, more than one generation is affected. A thorough family history may identify other family members who had similar types of vascular lesions. At this point, most vascular malformations do not have an identifiable genetic cause, although scientists are avidly investigating the potential genetic basis of these disorders and identifying new mutations every year.

Researchers have studied family patterns and identified certain genetic mutations associated with the affected individuals. Mutations of the following genes have been linked to familial vascular malformations: Tie-2, **RASA-1**, Glomulin, flt-4 (lymphatic), endoglin, ALK-1, and others. These genes play a role in various aspects of normal vascular development. If a patient is suspected of having a vascular anomaly for which a genetic mutation has been identified, blood samples from the patient and parents can be sent to laboratories studying these. Currently, the genetic testing for **hereditary hemorrhagic telangiectasia** (also known as Osler Weber Rendu), is the only approved (i.e., nonresearch) test for a genetic mutation associated with vascular anomalies (Figure 12). The initial testing is for mutations of endoglin or ALK-1. Once a mutation is identified, other family members can be easily screened for that mutation.

Your physician can discuss how genetic testing for other vascular malformations can be undertaken. A consultation with a genetics specialist and genetic counselor may also be recommended. Additionally, you or your child may be eligible for research projects in which blood

RASA-1

RAS p21 protein activator (GTPase activating protein) 1, CMAVM; CM-AVM

Hereditary hemorrhagic telangiectasia

Familial condition with multifocal arteriovenous malformations on mucosal surfaces (nasal passages, lips, gastrointestinal tract) and/or the brain, lungs, and liver.

Vascular Malformations

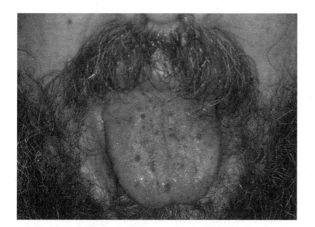

Figure 12   Hereditary hemorrhagic telangiectasia (HHT).

samples are collected for genetic studies. Table 1 lists genetic mutations that have been identified in vascular malformations to date.

33. If my child has a vascular malformation, does that mean there may be others?

Sometimes a vascular malformation extends beyond what is obvious. For this reason, the radiologic studies (often MRI) will include nearby structures. For example, a patient with a vascular malformation of the leg may have an MRI to study not only the leg but also the chest, abdomen, pelvis, and sometimes the brain.

Finding more extensive involvement is important as a baseline; however, in most cases, additional anomalies are not identified, and not all vascular malformations that are identified are symptomatic.

34. Are vascular malformations affected by hormonal changes?

Yes, vascular malformations may be responsive to hormonal changes. Some vascular anomalies are present at birth but often do not become apparent until years later, often during puberty. Hormonal changes related to puberty, pregnancy, and menopause can cause a vascular malformation to grow. In fact, even the hormonal changes related to a woman's menstrual cycle can cause slight growth or changes to a vascular malformation. For example, a woman may notice slight swelling or mild discomfort in a vascular lesion around the time of her period.

35. Can there be vascular malformations in the brain?

There are several vascular malformations that may affect the vessels of the brain. Some of these are diagnosed prenatally or shortly after birth, such as the

vein of Galen malformation. Vein of Galen malformation is a type of arteriovenous malformation involving the vein of Galen. Emergency embolization may be necessary to control high-output cardiac failure if it does not respond to medical management. There is a risk of bleeding from any intracranial arteriovenous malformation, and if this occurs, there is a high mortality and morbidity (permanent deficits) rate; therefore, once the diagnosis is made, treatment is recommended if possible. Treatment is often **endovascular therapy** (i.e., angiogram with embolization, insertion of coils or other agents into the abnormal vessel) or surgery. Vascular malformations of the brain may first be diagnosed after a seizure, a hemorrhage, a stroke, localized neurologic deficits without stroke, an excruciating headache, vision disturbances, or memory lapses, or diagnosis may occur incidentally without symptoms. Immediate evaluation is necessary for diagnosis and appropriate treatment.

Patients with arteriovenous malformations (Figure 13) often experience a "swishing" noise or sensation.

Dural fistulas occur when there is an abnormal connection between the blood vessels of the covering of the brain, the *dura mater*. A fistula is an aberrant, or abnormal,

Vein of galen malformation

Structural malformation of an embryonic cerebral vein resulting in high flow arteriovenous shunting of blood—can result in neonatal high-output cardiac failure, stroke, hydrocephalus, and/or neurological deficits.

Endovascular therapy

Treatment within the vessel via a catheter.

Vascular Malformations

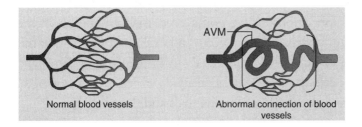

Figure 13   Arteriovenous malformation depicting abnormal connection of blood vessels. Adapted from: Randall T, Higashida. What is an arteriovenous malformation (AVM)? From the Cerebrovascular Imaging and Intervention Committee of the American Heart Association Cardiovascular Council.

connection between an artery and a vein. There are several types of dural fistulas, depending on their location. Most common types are the following:

- *Carotid cavernous sinus dural fistulas* occur behind the eye, triggering ophthalmologic symptoms from augmented blood flow to the orbit. Patients have eye swelling, decreased vision, double vision, redness, and congestion of the eye.
- *Transverse-sigmoid sinus dural fistulas* occur behind the ear, causing headache, neck pain, and/or a blood flow sound in parallel with the heartbeat (a bruit). Seizure or hemorrhage can occur if there is blood flow from the malformation to the vein of the brain.
- *Superior sagittal sinus dural fistulas* occur toward the top of the head in the midline, leading to similar symptoms.

Helpful Web sites for further information include:

- American Stroke Association (Search for the term "AVM.")
- Brain and Spine Foundation (See the online guide "Vascular Malformations of the Brain.")

Many patients are curious to know if vascular anomalies of the brain are genetic. Patients with hereditary hemorrhagic telangiectasia may have intracerebral arteriovenous malformations. Cavernoma-type malformations of the brain vessels may also occur in families, in which case the lesions are often multifocal. In both of these disorders, mutations have been identified, which permits genetic screening of affected individuals and their families.

RASA-1 mutations have been identified in many patients with cranial arteriovenous malformations. Characteristically, these patients also have many localized flat red/pink capillary malformations on the body surface.

36. Can vascular anomalies be diagnosed prenatally (before birth)?

Sometimes vascular malformations are diagnosed prenatally by ultrasound and fetal MRI. Asymmetric limbs and/or high-flow lesions may be spotted this way. Also large cysts seen in lymphatic malformations may be detected prenatally.

Sometimes vascular malformations are diagnosed prenatally by ultrasound and fetal MRI.

Prenatal diagnosis may allow for medical/surgical in utero intervention before the baby is born. For example, a large hepatic hemangioma causing high blood flow may be treated in utero by having the mother take certain medications. High-flow RICH-type hemangiomas have also been managed by maternal ingestion of digoxin or other medications, which cross the placenta and in turn treat the fetus. Some large vascular anomalies (e.g., large lesions that may compromise the airway) may require careful preparation for delivery.* Rarely, fetal surgery is performed to avert a life-threatening situation.

37. What risks are associated with anesthesia, especially for children?

Modern anesthesia performed by experienced anesthesiologists is much less risky than in the past. Risks will vary depending on the extent of the procedure, the location and nature of the problem, and any associated conditions. Often the child's pediatrician will be required to provide "medical clearance" in anticipation of anesthesia.

---

*Sometimes the EXIT procedure (ex utero intrapartum treatment procedure) is necessary, whereby the infant is partially delivered via cesarean section, remaining attached by the umbilical cord until physicians establish a stable airway. This procedure requires a specially trained team of physicians, nurses, and ancillary medical staff. Identification of a large extremity or vascular mass may also indicate a cesarean section delivery.

Vascular Malformations

Additionally, other specialists (e.g., cardiologist, otolaryngologist, endocrinologist) will need to provide clearance as well. If the child has been on steroid treatment, stress dosing for the anesthesia may be required. It is best to discuss any questions with the involved physicians ahead of time.

Susan and Ken say:

Our doctor recommended that our daughter get an MRI. Because she was only 4 months old at the time, she was going to have to receive general anesthesia in order to do the MRI, and we were very worried about the risks associated with anesthesia in such a young child. We hesitated and stalled getting an MRI for a couple of weeks because we thought that having to "put our baby under" general anesthesia posed a greater risk than the growth of an internal hemangioma. At the suggestion of our doctor, we spoke in advance to the anesthesiologist, who was able to allay our fears. Although you can never totally eliminate anesthesia risk, in the hands of an experienced doctor who has administered anesthesia to many children, we felt that the risks were extremely low, and in the end, we were glad she got the MRI.

38. When can blood clots form in a vascular malformation?

Due to sluggish blood flow through abnormal veins, clots may form in vascular malformations. This will occur more frequently if a person is immobilized (e.g., bedridden), when legs are crossed (which stifles blood flow), and if there is an underlying hematologic predisposition to thrombose (clot). If there is a poorly developed deep venous system, then even blood clots in superficial veins may be clinically significant.

If a blood clot is small and in a superficial vein, it may feel like a small pea and feel tender for several days.

The pain often responds to Advil or Motrin. Deeper clots are treated with anticoagulation therapy. Generally, heparin or low-molecular-weight heparin (LMWH) is initiated. LMWH is administered via injection into the subcutaneous tissue twice daily. The dose is based on the patient's weight. Some patients are transitioned to Coumadin, an oral medication. This drug requires more frequent blood testing. Newer oral anticoagulants that require less monitoring have been studied and will likely be on the market in the near future. See Question 24 for information about phleboliths.

39. Can women take birth control pills when they have a vascular malformation?

It is recommended that estrogen-containing birth control pills be avoided in women with vascular malformations, as unwanted blood clots can develop. Since birth control pills can be prescribed for a number of indications including irregular periods, acne, and hirsutism (extra unwanted hair growth), your doctor may discuss the potential side effects of birth control pills when your child is an early adolescent. Other forms of birth control are recommended.

40. Can a woman become pregnant and support a pregnancy when she has a vascular malformation?

In general, a woman who has a vascular malformation should be monitored closely during pregnancy and followed by a specialist in maternal fetal medicine, as many cases will be considered high-risk pregnancies and will warrant close monitoring of the mother and fetus.

Even women with large vascular malformations of the legs and pelvis have undergone successful pregnancies;

however, they benefit from being followed by an obstetrician familiar with patients who have complex medical issues. Women with vascular malformations may be treated with aspirin therapy or low-molecular-weight heparin (**Lovenox**) to prevent excessive blood clotting. Even with treatment, affected pregnant women may experience swelling of the vascular malformation, legs, vulva, and varicose veins of the legs.

Lovenox

Agent administered subcutaneously to prevent further blood clots; brand name for Enoxaparin injection.

41. What are some medications used to treat patients with vascular malformations?

There is no medication that will "cure" a vascular malformation, although current management can result in clinical success and complete radiologic eradication of the malformations. Clinical trials are up and coming for those malformations that behave aggressively and cause complications such as skeletal deformities, bleeding disorders, pain, and organ damage.

Medications are generally prescribed on an as-needed basis to manage pain, infection, bleeding, or clotting. Procedures may also be recommended to improve or to prevent problems.

New research trials are in the pipeline, using medications to inhibit unwanted symptoms associated with vascular malformations, for the most challenging vascular malformations associated with progressive symptoms.

Susan and Ken say:

Our daughter was put on prednisolone at 4 months old to treat multiple facial hemangiomas. She was on prednisolone for 1 month, and after seeing very little progress, our doctor switched her to propranolol. Within only 24 hours, we saw substantial improvement, which has continued in the last few months. We feel very lucky that she reacted so well to the propranolol. There is no way to be sure how anyone will react to a particular medication, and you have to prepare yourself for the fact that it may take some time to find the right one for your child.

42. What are the risks of not having a vascular malformation treated?

Some vascular malformations do not require intervention and can be managed through observation. For other vascular malformations, treatment will help alleviate pain or discomfort, limb length and girth discrepancies, and psychosocial stigmata. With treatment, the lesions may be greatly improved, and if they are not cured they may be greatly improved functionally and cosmetically.

For patients with "aggressive" vascular malformations— a scenario that often arises in the peripubertal years—it may seem frustrating to only treat symptoms as they develop. Until we have improved medical therapies, however, symptomatic intervention is advised.

PART THREE

Facts About Hemangiomas

What are some of the different kinds
of hemangiomas?

Are certain people more likely to
have hemangiomas?

When is surgery recommended to treat
hemangiomas, and what are the possible
complications?

More . . .

43. What causes hemangiomas?

Hemangiomas are caused by overgrowths of endothelial cells, but scientists do not understand exactly why this happens. Although there is no definitive or unified theory, research indicates hemangiomas may be due to a number of influences: hormonal, mechanical, environmental, and genetic.

44. What are some of the different kinds of hemangiomas?

Two main categories of hemangiomas include *congenital* and *infantile* hemangiomas.

Congenital hemangiomas are completely formed at birth and may be detected through ultrasound before birth. They can be classified further based on their ability to involute, or spontaneously shrink, as either NICH (noninvoluting congenital hemangiomas) or RICH (rapidly involuting congenital hemangiomas).

Infantile hemangiomas usually become noticeable and/or start to grow in the first few weeks after birth and are the most common type of hemangioma. In fact, infantile hemangiomas are the most common type of noncancerous tumor. Usually these lesions have a very characteristic pattern of growing rapidly, often for up to a year after birth, stabilizing, and then spontaneously shrinking (or involuting).

A growth curve illustrating the natural course of typical hemangiomas, RICH and NICH, is shown in Figure 14.

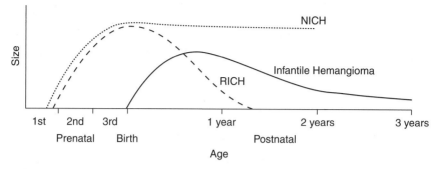

Figure 14   Hemangioma growth curve. Adapted from: Mulliken JB, Enjolras O. Congenital hemangiomas and infantile hemangioma: missing links. *J Am Acad Dermatol*. June 2004; 50(6):875–82.

Hemangiomas may be further classified according to the extent of involved tissue as follows:

- Superficial (capillary or venular hemangiomas or strawberry mark)
- Deep (hemangiomas without a superficial red component)
- Combined (mixed hemangiomas)
- Segmental (diffuse or regional hemangiomas)

45. What is hemangiomatosis?

Hemangiomatosis is the term for when there are several small hemangiomas on the skin and/or internal organs. Symptoms range from none to severe.

When a child has several hemangiomas visible on the skin, the first step is usually a careful physical examination. An abdominal ultrasound should be performed in search of hemangiomas in the liver or elsewhere in the abdomen. The child should also be monitored for blood in the stool or any other symptoms. Some physicians perform an ultrasound of the head as well. If the ultrasound

Facts About Hemangiomas

studies are normal, none of the hemangiomas are in alarming locations, and the child remains asymptomatic, feeding well and acting normally for age, the child is monitored. See Question 73 for more about the management of liver hemangiomas.

46. Are hemangiomas painful?

In general, hemangiomas are not painful. However, if the surface is ulcerated, this can cause discomfort. Sometimes ulcerations can be quite extensive and severe. They can also become infected or bleed. There are a number of ways to manage these types of complications, and it is best to discuss this with the treating physician. Hemangiomas may be itchy if the surface is dry and scaly and also during the involution phase. Parents are advised to keep the child's nails short to prevent undue irritation of the hemangioma.

47. Are certain people more likely to have hemangiomas?

Hemangiomas can occur in any child; however, they occur more frequently in females, babies born prematurely, and multiples (twins or triplets). They occur more commonly in the head and neck region, and they are uncommon in very dark-skinned individuals.

Researchers are trying to identify the potential causes, including genetic reasons, that hemangiomas develop.

48. Are hemangiomas inherited, and do genetics play a role?

Rarely, hemangiomas affect multiple generations in one family. More often, they occur "sporadically," with a relatively high incidence, occurring in up to 13% of newborns. Researchers are trying to identify the potential causes, including genetic reasons, that hemangiomas develop.

49. Do adults get hemangiomas?

Strictly speaking, *hemangioma* refers only to the type of vascular lesion occurring in infants. Even so, medical reports state older children and adults have hemangiomas of the liver, spine, or brain when in fact these are vascular malformations, usually venous. Similarly, pathology reports often describe vascular malformations, yet the final diagnosis is listed as hemangioma. This may lead to confusion, as true hemangiomas are those that have the typical life cycle seen in infancy, and these spontaneously involute. If an adult has a "true" hemangioma, it is the residual tissue after involution of a hemangioma of infancy. Sometimes parents will show a residual hemangioma to the child's physician.

50. If my child has a hemangioma, does that mean there are hemangiomas in other locations?

Having one hemangioma does not indicate there are multiple hemangiomas in other locations. In general, if five or more hemangiomas of the skin are present, further studies will be performed to screen for hemangiomas elsewhere. Usually the first screening test is an ultrasound. Additionally, if there are any clinical symptoms present to suggest the presence of other hemangiomas, tests will be recommended.

Susan and Ken say:

Our child was born with hemangiomas in front of both ears, on her lips, and inside her mouth. Our doctor advised us that it is very possible that she might have other hemangiomas in other locations, including inside her body. Because hers were all on her face, we were told that there was a somewhat higher probability that she might have one in her throat. Our doctor suggested that we see an ear, nose, and throat specialist, who was very helpful in determining that she probably did not have one in her throat, but let us know what the warning signs are of an internal airway hemangioma that is growing.

51. What is a "segmental" hemangioma?

A segmental hemangioma is one that follows a certain anatomic distribution, as depicted in Figure 15. Studies have shown that certain segmental hemangiomas, especially those on the face, can be associated with other medical issues, such as PHACES association.

52. What is a RICH?

RICH is an acronym for **r**apidly **i**nvoluting **c**ongenital **h**emangioma (Figure 16). These hemangiomas are unusual in that they grew in utero, can be large at birth, and then gradually decrease in size. In contrast, typical hemangiomas do not grow in utero but instead grow after birth then spontaneously involute. RICH lesions may

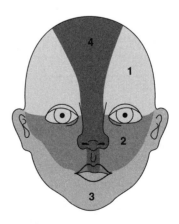

Figure 15 **Segmental patterns associated with a segmental hemangioma. Adapted from:** *Pediatrics.* **2006; 117(3):699.**

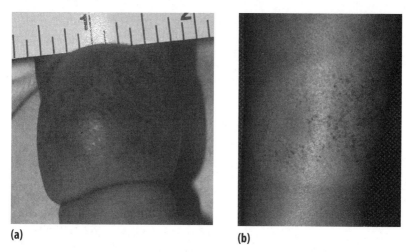

(a)   (b)

Figure 16   Hemangiomas: (a) RICH-type hemangioma before treatment; (b) RICH-type hemangioma after treatment.

be symptomatic in utero, due to high blood flow within the lesion. They also may be quite large, which could influence the type of delivery.

53. Do RICH-type hemangiomas cause any problems?

Occasionally, RICH lesions have large feeding arteries and can cause a strain on the heart in utero or shortly after birth. This type of RICH will require medical therapy and possibly embolization. There also may be some abnormal blood tests such as low platelet count during the first week of life, which may warrant treatment. These abnormalities are not as severe as seen in Kasabach-Merritt phenomenon (see Figure 19 in Question 72); however, making the diagnosis of a RICH-type lesion is not always easy.

Jessica says:

Our son's RICH did cause some problems for him. As we understood it, the clotting factors in his blood were being pulled to the affected area. He required a few platelet transfusions.

Also, at 5 days old, the hemangioma started bleeding and it took a while for it to stop. That was the point we realized we may have a serious problem on our hands. This prompted an immediate embolization.

54. What diagnostic blood tests are commonly used, and what information do they provide?

A listing of common blood tests related to the diagnosis and treatment of hemangiomas is shown in Table 6.

55. I heard about GLUT-1 as a marker for hemangiomas. What is this?

GLUT-1 stands for glucose transporter type 1, which is a molecule present on the surface of typical hemangioma tissues. It is not present on vascular malformations. Since GLUT-1 is also present on placenta cells, there is speculation that some hemangiomas may be due to placental tissue that dislodged and relocated to the fetus, later becoming a hemangioma.

Table 6   Blood Tests for Patients with Hemangiomas

Test	What Information Does the Test Provide?	Who is Evaluated?
T_4, TSH	Thyroid function	Patients with liver hemangiomas and patients requiring PHACES evaluation
Complete blood count (CBC)	White cell count, red cell count, platelet count	Patients with bleeding hemangiomas, suspected Kasabach-Merritt phenomenon, or RICH
Coagulation profile, fibrinogen, fibrin degradation products, D-dimers	Clotting profile; assessment for breakdown products of clotting, which may be seen in "activated" endothelium of certain vascular anomalies	
Liver function, alpha-fetoprotein (AFP)	Synthetic function of liver, liver enzymes, tumor marker (AFP)	Patients with hepatic (liver) hemangiomas

56. Why is observation the preferred treatment for some hemangiomas?

Most hemangiomas are harmless and often resolve on their own without any treatment. Hemangiomas usually appear within the first few weeks of life. Although they can grow very rapidly, at about 6–12 months hemangiomas often involute or shrink spontaneously (Figure 17). Hemangiomas that are fully developed at birth are likely to involute even sooner. Many hemangiomas shrink completely by the time a child is 3 to 4 years of age, however there may be remaining signs (such as stretched out or discolored skin with an irregular contour) which can be improved with surgical or other interventions. Once hemangiomas shrink, they will not reoccur.

Many doctors prefer observation, or "watchful waiting," because the chances are very good that a hemangioma will resolve on its own with few, if any, side effects or treatment complications. This also depends on the

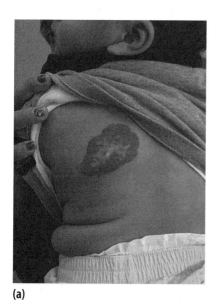

(a)

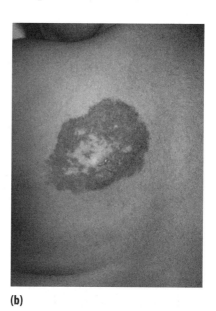

(b)

Figure 17 Hemangiomas: (a) hemangioma with early involution; (b) hemongioma with late involution.

All hemangiomas, however, including hemangiomas of infancy, should be evaluated and followed by an experienced doctor who can determine the right treatment approach.

location of the hemangioma, as not all hemangiomas involute perfectly. In some cases, medical or laser/surgical interventions in early infancy may preclude the need for more involved procedures when the child is older.

All hemangiomas, however, should be evaluated and followed by an experienced doctor who can determine the right treatment approach. Some patients are at risk for serious medical complications that could include bleeding, ulceration, pain, infection, visual sequelae (**proptosis, ptosis, astigmatism, amblyopia**), and interrupted breathing. The American Academy of Dermatology recommends that *all* hemangiomas of infancy be evaluated for possible complications.

57. What are red flags I should be concerned about?

Most hemangiomas involute on their own and are not worrisome, but they are a cause for concern when they involve any of the following:

- *Airway*: Hemangiomas involving the airway or throat can cause breathing problems. If left untreated, rapid growth could cause obstructions or blockages to the airway.
- *Eyes*: Hemangiomas near an eye can cause astigmatism, ptosis, amblyopia, and other visual problems. With treatment, however, most visual problems resolve.
- *Spine/midline*: The spine and midline are also critical areas. Hemangiomas in the midline over the spine can cause neurologic problems.
- *Bleeding/ulcerating*: Ulcerating lesions are prone to infection and require medical care. Bleeding hemangiomas require medical and/or surgical attention.
- *Large, segmental hemangiomas*: Lesions presenting in this pattern require evaluation for PHACES association, which may suggest a variety of other medical issues.

Proptosis

Prominent or bulging eyes; can be due to mass (e.g., hemangioma or vascular malformation) pushing the eyeball forward.

Ptosis

Drooping upper eyelid that may cover the eye's pupil.

Astigmatism

Vision defect that is caused by changes to curvature of the cornea; vision can be blurred and/or distorted.

Amblyopia

Poor vision in one eye (rarely both eyes) due to deficient visual stimulation in early childhood, especially infancy.

58. Why are corticosteroids prescribed to treat hemangiomas?

Corticosteroids are often the first course of treatment for hemangiomas. In fact, the majority of hemangiomas respond well to corticosteroid treatment. Depending on a hemangioma's size and location, corticosteroids can be administered orally, by injection into the lesion, or topically on the skin's surface. Exactly how corticosteroids work in this case is not known, but improved color from red to iridescent/grayish is often the first sign of steroid response. These findings are also seen with natural involution. The medication speeds up the process.

Corticosteroids are *not* the same as anabolic steroids, which are used illegally to enhance athletic performance. However, corticosteroids are strong medications and do have side effects that should be discussed with your doctor. Corticosteroids generally are *not* effective in treating other types of vascular anomalies.

Common names of oral steroids used to treat hemangiomas include prednisone, Prelone, Orapred, and prednisolone. Triamcinolone acetate and betamethasone sodium phosphate (or acetate) are corticosteroids commonly given by injection (**intralesionally**) directly into some hemangiomas.

Corticosteroids
Class of steroid drugs often used to treat inflammation, swelling, and/or pain.

Intralesional
Into the lesion; for example, intralesional injection of a medication.

59. What are some of the possible side effects of corticosteroids, especially among young children? Can my child attend day care while he or she is taking corticosteroids?

Corticosteroids are commonly used to treat a variety of health problems by reducing inflammation and influencing the immune system. Corticosteroids are often prescribed for a short time period and require an increasingly lower (or tapered) dose near the end of treatment.

Facts About Hemangiomas

Possible side effects for short-term use include:

- Irritability, behavior changes, trouble sleeping
- Increased appetite
- Puffy, chubby face
- Indigestion, upset stomach
- Acne, baby acne
- Pubic hair growth (even in young children)
- Sluggish linear growth, developmental delays due to chubbiness
- **Immunosuppression**, reduced ability to fight infection

Immunosuppression
Prevention of the body's natural immune response.

Because steroids reduce the body's ability to fight infection, it would be best to reduce the risk of situations that expose a child on treatment to the flu, colds, viruses, infection, pinkeye, and chickenpox. Obviously, not every family is able to avoid day care during treatment. Emphasizing positive hygiene habits such as hand washing, helping your child avoid playing with sick children, and using your best judgment will help enormously.

There have been reports of infants on steroids developing a lung infection caused by *Pneumocystis carinii*. This illness can be prevented by prophylactic doses of an antibiotic (e.g., Septra, Bactrim) given twice daily 2 or 3 days per week.

Because behavior changes and irritability that result from steroid treatment may affect your child's social interactions, it may be helpful to inform babysitters, day care workers, and other adults in charge that your child is being treated with corticosteroids.

Susan and Ken say:

Our doctor took us through all of the possible side effects of corticosteroids in young children, and listening to the long list is intimidating and discouraging. It is important to remember that the overwhelming majority of kids do not experience any of these side effects, and most of the side effects stop when you stop using the medicine. (We feel fortunate that like most children, our daughter did not experience any side effects.)

Jeannine says:

Our daughter started prednisone when she was 1 month old and was tapered off by the time she was 9 months old. We were very fortunate that she did not experience any extreme side affects from the corticosteroid therapy. The side effects that she did experience were limited to a chubby baby face and some occasional irritability. On those occasions where it was difficult to settle or calm her down, I would place her in a warm bath and bathe her. Almost immediately she would relax and be cooing and laughing once again. It worked every time!

60. What is interferon alfa-2a or interferon alfa-2b?

Interferon alfa is another drug that is sometimes used to treat hemangiomas when other medications are not effective. This drug is a type of immunotherapy, or biologic therapy that makes use of chemicals that occur naturally in the body. Interferon alfa is produced naturally by the body's white cells (lymphocytes) when they detect tumor growth. Interferon alfa has anti-angiogenic properties that inhibit new blood vessel growth and reduce cell growth.

Interferon alfa is administered via injection. It is rarely used for hemangiomas and, if so, only after other therapies have failed, as there may be significant neurologic side effects associated with its use in young infants (Table 7). Kaposiform hemangioendotheliomas may respond to interferon alfa therapy as well.

Table 7   Medications for Vascular Anomalies

Medications for Hemangiomas	Route of Administration	Possible Mechanism of Action	Potential Side Effects

Corticosteroids
  Orapred (prednisolone)
  Temovate (clobetasol propionate)
  Ultravate
  Kenalog
	Oral
	
	Topical
	
	Intralesional
		Vasoconstriction
		
		Slows progression of hemangioma growth
		
		Induces involution
			Weight gain, immune suppression, irritability, adrenal suppression, hypertension

Interferon alfa	Subcutaneous	Slows progression of hemangioma growth Induces involution Anti-angiogenic	Liver dysfunction, neurologic symptoms, blood count changes
Propranolol	Oral	Vasoconstriction of hemangioma	Low blood pressure, constipation, low blood sugar
Vincristine	Intravenous (via surgically inserted IV catheter)		Constipation, nerve damage Pain or redness at injection site if accidentally infused into surrounding tissue
Medications for Hemangioendothelioma	**Route of Administration**	**Action**	**Potential Side Effects**
Corticosteroids	Intralesional Topical Oral Intravenous	Vasoconstriction Anti-angiogenic	Immune suppression See above
Vincristine	Intravenous (through indwelling catheter)	Anti-angiogenic	See above
Amicar	Oral	Prevents dissolution of clot	Increased blood clotting

Table 7   Medications for Vascular Anomalies (*Continued*)

Medications for vascular/lymphatic malformations	Route of Administration	Possible Mechanism of Action	Potential Side Effects
Aspirin, Advil, Motrin	Oral	Anti-inflammatory, antiplatelet effect	Bleeding
Lovenox (low-molecular-weight heparin)	Subcutaneous injection	Prevents blood clots	Pain at site of administration, bleeding
Coumadin (warfarin)	Oral	Prevents blood clots	Dose sensitive to diet, other medications; requires frequent blood tests to monitor effect; bleeding
Bleomycin (for sclerotherapy)	Intralesional	Causes inflammation within sac of malformation	Lung damage if systemic absorption
Doxycycline	Intralesional	Causes inflammation within sac of malformation	Tooth staining if systemic absorption in early childhood
Picibanil	Intralesional	Causes inflammation within sac of malformation	Contraindicated if allergic to penicillin

61. How is laser therapy used to treat complicated hemangiomas?

Flashlamp pulsed dye laser therapy may be effective in preventing outward growth of hemangiomas. The laser targets hemoglobin in the red blood cells, lessening the color of the hemangioma. A series of treatments are required. Laser therapy may be used in conjunction with medical therapy, and the results may be impressive.

Facts About Hemangiomas

Laser therapy may improve ulcerated hemangiomas. Additionally, laser therapy may be used after involution of a hemangioma to eradicate residual vessels on the surface of the skin. Different types of laser therapy can smooth the contour of the skin, which may improve the skin's surface, especially scarring that was caused by ulcerations. Other types of lasers may be used for hemangiomas in the airway (**subglottic hemangiomas**).

62. When is surgery recommended to treat hemangiomas, and what are the possible complications?

In general, surgeons prefer to delay intervention for hemangiomas, as an excellent cosmetic and functional result is likely to occur naturally.

In general, surgeons prefer to delay intervention for hemangiomas, as an excellent cosmetic and functional result is likely to occur naturally. Surgically removing a hemangioma may help in situations that include large scalp hemangiomas or visually occlusive, ulcerated, infected, or bleeding hemangiomas that do not respond to medical therapy. In some instances, early surgical therapy is preferable to other therapies. Later surgical therapy (i.e., after the hemangioma has involuted) is often required to remove residual scarring, thin or sagging skin, or bulkiness, and to improve the aesthetic result.

It is important to note that not every hemangioma is the same and not every physician treats hemangiomas the same. Different physicians may have varying opinions about the best approach.

63. What is propranolol, and how is it used for treatment?

While **propranolol** has been used for many years for the treatment of high blood pressure, in 2008 it was serendipitously noted to improve hemangiomas when this medication was prescribed (for a cardiac indication) to a child who had a hemangioma. Physicians are still learning how best to administer and monitor propranolol therapy in infants with hemangiomas, and preliminary reports seem promising.

Pediatric cardiologists have prescribed this medication for many years for infants and children with cardiac disorders; thus they have had more experience with propranolol. As with steroid treatment, rebound hemangioma growth can be seen after discontinuing the medication, so resuming therapy (albeit at a lower dose) may be necessary.

Propranolol and other medications used for medical therapy of hemangiomas are used "off-label"—that is, there has been no study for this therapy approved by the U.S. Food and Drug Administration (FDA), and the product labeling does not indicate its use for hemangiomas. Since the original publication describing propranolol and hemangiomas, several other reports have documented successful use of this therapy. Caution must always be exercised, and potential side effects (such as low blood sugar, low blood pressure) as well as unforeseen complications must be discussed.

Susan and Ken say:

When our daughter's hemangiomas were not improving in response to the corticosteroids, our doctor suggested that she try propranolol. Because the use of propranolol for hemangioma is very new and "off-label," we were wary of giving it to our daughter. We were worried that there would be some side effects that would show up later in her life, given that it is being used for an alternative purpose. We ended up speaking to many doctors, from hemangioma specialists to cardiologists, as well as other parents whose children had been taking it. We were comforted by the fact that propranolol itself is not a new medicine and the doctors we spoke with told us that it was considered a very safe medication for heart-related treatments. In addition, the parents whose children were taking propranolol for hemangiomas had achieved such dramatic results that we thought it was worth trying. We are thankful that our daughter has responded so well to the propranolol with no side effects.

64. What is vincristine, and how is it used for treatment?

Vincristine

Type of chemotherapy drug given by injection into a vein (often an indwelling intravenous line such as a mediport or Broviac catheter is required); sometimes used for hemangiomas.

Vincristine is a chemotherapy drug that was first approved by the FDA in 1963 for the primary use of treating patients with cancer. Vincristine belongs to a class of drugs known as vinca alkaloids and works by interrupting rapidly growing cells, such as those of a proliferative hemangioma, and "programming" those cells to die (apoptosis). Complex hemangiomas that are fast growing and unresponsive to steroid or propranolol treatment may respond to vincristine.

Mediport

Indwelling intravenous access device inserted surgically facilitating blood drawing and permitting safe administration of fluids, blood products, and medications, preventing leakage to outside tissues.

Vincristine (brand name Oncovin) is given through an intravenous (IV) infusion through a permanently placed catheter such as a **mediport** or **broviac catheter**, which is inserted surgically under general anesthesia. Parents must discuss with the child's physician the possible side effects of vincristine. As a chemotherapy drug, it can reduce the body's immune response and can cause low white blood cell (neutrophil) counts, or neutropenia, which puts a person at risk for infection and illness. Vincristine is not routinely used as a first-line therapy, as there are other alternatives (e.g., steroids and propranolol, both given orally). If there is limited or no response to the oral therapies, or if a patient is unable to be treated with the others, vincristine should be considered.

65. How are childhood immunizations affected by the treatment of a child's hemangioma?

Parents of young children with hemangiomas should make plans to suspend their children's live virus immunizations if they are being treated with corticosteroids. During the first year of life, the only live virus vaccine that is routinely administered is the rotavirus vaccine. Other live virus vaccinations are given at 1 year of age (varicella vaccine) and 15 months of age (measles, mumps, rubella vaccine). Steroid therapy, which suppresses the immune response, may lead to an increased susceptibility to the infection. Other non-live virus vaccinations may be administered. Ideally, the first set of immunizations (due at 2 months of age) would be administered at least 2 weeks prior to the initiation of steroid therapy. While steroids will not be dangerous, they will depress the immune response the vaccinations aim to produce. All subsequent immunizations are booster doses that heighten the initial immune response, which is the most essential. Of note, use of propranolol does not seem to affect the immune system.

Patients over 6 months of age as well as family members should receive the influenza vaccine. Infants with airway hemangiomas may benefit from the respiratory synctitial virus (RSV) vaccination series (Synagis™—palivizumab).

66. What should someone do if they are exposed to chickenpox during steroid treatment?

Your medical team needs to know if any member of the family has been exposed to or develops varicella (chickenpox virus). If a child on steroids is exposed to a contagious individual, he or she may develop a more severe form of the disease. Immune globulin treatment may be required for exposure, and prompt institution of antiviral therapy will be required if varicella develops.

67. Why is my child's hemangioma bleeding/ulcerating?

Researchers do not know exactly what causes a hemangioma to ulcerate, but ulceration is very common. In fact, it is the most common complication of hemangiomas and is most likely to occur in mucosal areas such as the lip, vagina, and rectal areas. When a hemangioma is ulcerating, the disruption to the epithelial lining makes it more likely to bleed or become infected, which may be extremely painful. If in the oral area, the ulceration can affect feeding; if it is in the diaper area, infants may withhold stooling due to pain. Ulcerated hemangiomas are also likely to scar.

Jessica says:

Our son's hemangioma started ulcerating. There were large open sores which formed in a few places. It was extremely important for the area to stay clean, which was hard since it was on his buttocks. Often stool would touch the area—however, no problems surfaced because of it. The ulcerations actually looked very serious, but the doctor assured us that they were part of the healing process and would eventually go away, which they did.

68. How are ulcerated hemangiomas treated?

Hemangiomas in certain parts of the body are more likely to ulcerate, especially in the following areas:

Perineum

Area between the anus and external genitalia.

- Mucosal areas such as the lip or, **perineum**, rectum
- Areas where the skin is likely to chafe
- Pressure point areas such as the back or buttock

It is very important for an ulcerated hemangioma to be evaluated and treated promptly by a doctor to prevent infection (Figure 18). Ulcerated hemangiomas may respond to basic wound care treatment such as antibiotic cream, Vaseline gauze, or hydrocolloid gels. They should be kept as clean as possible.

Infected lesions will require antibiotic treatment, sometimes administered topically into the lesion (locally) and other times an oral antibiotic is prescribed. Sometimes other therapies may be needed such as steroids, propranolol, or flashlamp pulsed dye laser therapy.

Pain can be managed by topical or oral pain medications. Discomfort can also be relieved by simple techniques such as sitz baths several times per day, air drying, and using foam cushions with areas cut out to relieve pressure from the affected area. Be prepared for your doctor to try several different trial and error approaches before noticing a response to treatment.

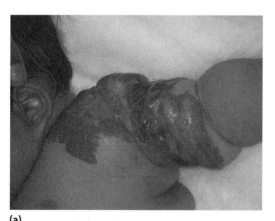
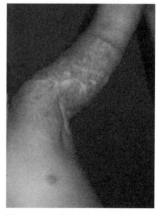

(a)   (b)

Figure 18   Hemangiomas: (a) ulcerated hemangioma before treatment; (b) ulcerated hemangioma after treatment.

Jessica says:

Based solely on physical appearance, the ulcerations were the worst part of the condition. We had to clean the area with sterile saline, iodine, bacitracin, and sterile gauze. Each time a diaper change was needed, an entire cleaning ritual took place. It was completely necessary. Daunting but manageable, we figured out a whole routine that made it easy.

69. The doctor wants to evaluate my child for PHACES. What is that?

PHACES is an acronym for a constellation of findings associated with a segmental hemangioma, usually of the face (Table 8). A patient is considered to have PHACES if one or more of the features are present along with the hemangioma:

Posterior fossa abnormalities (structural abnormality of the brain)

Hemangiomas in a segmental distribution

Arterial anomalies of the brain, neck, or chest—can be abnormal branching of arteries, absent arteries, structurally abnormal vessels (corkscrew shaped, narrow, thin, dilated)

Cardiac anomalies—any structural abnormality of the heart

Eye abnormalities—glaucoma, iris, retina, cornea abnormalities including cataracts

Sternal or other midline anomalies and/or spinal axis involvement—sternal bone anomalies or absence of the sternum; skin tags over the midline of the chest; abnormal thyroid function; clefting of the lip, palate, nose, or other midline structure; midabdominal "raphe" or vertical scarlike appendage above the umbilicus

Table 8   PHACES

Meaning of Acronym Letter	Examples
Posterior fossa or other structural abnormality in the brain	Dandy-Walker malformation of brain Cerebellar abnormalities
Hemangioma (segmental, usually on the face)	Cutaneous hemangioma, usually on the face, in a defined area following one or more "segmental" pattern noted in Figure 15.
Arterial abnormalities of the brain, neck or chest	Persistence of embryonic vessels Small, narrow arteries Abnormal branching of arteries Corkscrew appearance of arteries
Cardiac anomaly	Any structural anomaly of the heart or great vessels
Eye abnormalities not directly related to a hemangioma of the eye area	Cataract, glaucoma, abnormalities of the retina, iris
Sternal or other midline deformities	Absence of sternum Abnormalities of sternal bones Hypothyroidism Cleft lip/palate Midline skin tags or scarlike lesions over the sternum or above the umbilicus

70. Why is it so important to screen patients for PHACES?

Early detection of cardiac, endocrine (e.g., **hypothyroidism**), eye, or brain abnormalities are important, as sometimes medical or surgical intervention will be necessary. Furthermore, patients with PHACES need closer medical and radiologic monitoring and may be referred to other physicians such as a neurologist, neurosurgeon, or interventional neuroradiologist, if abnormalities of the brain or its vessels are detected.

Hypothyroidism

Condition of underactive thyroid gland, which can cause slowed metabolism and feelings of low energy.

Jeannine says:

Our daughter was born with a segmental hemangioma—a clue to her physician that it could mean a PHACES diagnosis for her. We were immediately sent off to meet with a pediatric ophthalmologist, where it was discovered that our daughter's hemangioma was on her iris. If we had not been advised to have her eye/vision evaluated, and the hemangioma was not discovered on her iris, our daughter could have lost the vision in her eye. Today, she has 20/20 vision!

Along with the ophthalmologist's evaluation, we were told that our daughter would also need a cardiac workup, as well as an MRI/MRA to screen for arterial/brain anomalies. Unfortunately both arterial/brain anomalies were found in our daughter, but we have learned that "knowledge is power"—never quite understood that until now. The best doctors in the field closely monitor her. I guess that is all we could ask for. She is a happy, smart, funny almost four-year-old little girl who is thriving. There is life after a diagnosis such as this . . . even happiness.

71. How are patients screened for PHACES?

Patients at risk for PHACES must undergo a thorough physical examination; blood tests (for thyroid function); an MRI of the brain (to evaluate the brain structure) and MRA of the brain, neck, and chest (for assessment of the arteries); cardiology evaluation with echocardiogram; radiologic assessment of the sternal bones; and thorough ophthalmologic evaluation.

Certainly if an infant has raspy breathing, an airway hemangioma should be promptly considered and evaluated.

Some patients with segmental hemangiomas of the lower face in the "beard" distribution are candidates for a PHACES evaluation as well as for hemangioma in the airway. These patients will require a screening examination by an otolaryngologist. Often patients with airway hemangiomas also have vascular staining of the soft palate, which can be a clue. Certainly if an infant has raspy breathing, an airway hemangioma should be promptly considered and evaluated.

If abnormalities consistent with the diagnosis of PHACES are identified, they must be followed closely. In conjunction with the PHACES evaluation, the hemangioma will likely be treated medically and possibly with flashlamp laser therapy as well.

72. The doctor says my child has kaposiform hemangioendothelioma (KHE). What is this?

KHE is a form of vascular anomaly that may be associated with a low platelet count, bleeding, coagulation test abnormalities and a red-purple, sometimes leathery, swollen area. These need to be treated with medications to prevent bleeding and other potential complications. Sometimes the physician can feel comfortable with the diagnosis by looking at it. Other times, a small piece of tissue must be removed (biopsied) and reviewed under the microscope.

Therapy for a kaposiform hemangioendothelioma may include steroids, vincristine, interferon alfa, surgery, embolization, compression, and antifibrinolytic medication (e.g., **aminocaproic acid**, which may improve the coagulopathy within the lesion). Kaposiform hemangioendothelioma may be severe and life-threatening, requiring prolonged hospitalization (for blood product support to prevent bleeding), observation, and medication (Figure 19). Other patients with kaposiform hemangioendothelioma experience lymphedema (swelling due to lymphatic vessel dilation within the lesion). This swelling may respond to lymphatic massage and compression therapy.

Aminocaproic acid
Medication prescribed to control bleeding problems when clots break down too quickly.

Sometimes kaposiform hemangioendothelioma is surgically removable; however, more commonly, the lesion "strands" into the musculature, making surgical excision difficult.

81

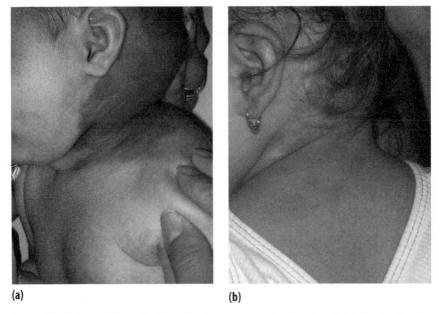

(a)   (b)

Figure 19   (a) KHE with Kasabach-Merritt phenomenon before treatment; (b) after treatment.

Carol says:

The hardest part of learning that my daughter had Kasabach–Merritt syndrome was now accepting and understanding the treatment she had to undergo. A 3-week-old, my angel, going through all of this medication and procedures was nonetheless necessary to save her life. First, a biopsy to confirm diagnosis. Now, the medication and transfusions. Since this tumor "eats" the platelets of the infant affected, platelet transfusions are common, necessary, and most of the time frequent, as well as blood transfusions. Chemotherapy—vincristine—was part of my daughter's treatment as well as medication to help with the coagulation. The treatment is aggressive and daily. It helps to ask questions and know what each medication is for and why it is needed.

73. My child has a liver hemangioma. Should I worry?

Not all liver hemangiomas are problematic. Many liver hemangiomas are symptom free and are monitored by frequent ultrasounds and follow-up by the treating physician. In severe cases, complications of liver hemangiomas include heart failure and thyroid problems, in which case medications and possible procedures will be recommended. Patients with this type of liver hemangioma have very large livers diffusely scattered with hemangiomas, causing high-output cardiac failure. The enlarged liver can compress other organs, causing **compartment syndrome**, and push the diaphragm upward, diminishing the lung volume and causing breathing difficulties. There are cases of severe forms of liver hemangiomas unresponsive to medical therapy that were treated successfully with liver transplantation.

It is important to note that adults are often told they have "liver hemangiomas," which are in fact hepatic vascular malformations, a common incidental finding and mistakenly called a hemangioma.

Compartment syndrome

Pressure on another organ, blood vessel, nerve, or other body part within a confined space.

Facts About Hemangiomas

PART FOUR

Lymphatic Malformations

What is a lymphatic malformation?

What precautions should I be aware of regarding lymphatic malformations?

What are some of the syndromes associated with lymphatic malformations?

More . . .

74. What is a lymphatic malformation?

Lymphatic malformations are abnormal growths of spongelike lymphatic vessels that transport lymphatic fluid. They create disruptions in flow of lymphatic fluid that cannot drain back into the bloodstream, causing lymph nodes and surrounding tissue to swell. Lymphatic malformations may be isolated or a collection of cysts filled with straw-colored fluid (lymph), or they may be more extensive and involve an extremity (arm or leg), the abdomen, or chest.

Lymphatic malformations occur early in embryonic development as the lymphatic system forms, usually by about 6 weeks. They occur due to small mistakes in cell division during this time of rapid growth and development. Animal models of **lymphedema** and lymphatic **dysplasia** as well as studies of cancer and lymphatic-dependent metastases have led to great strides in scientific research, unraveling essential pathways and modulators in lymphatic development. Nonetheless, there is a great lag in translating these findings into effective and novel means of treating lymphatic disorders.

Because lymph aids the body in fighting bacteria and the immune response, individuals may notice even more swelling of a lymphatic malformation when they are sick or receive immunizations. **Lymphangitis** is inflammation of lymphatic channels due to bacteria, fungi, viruses, and other organisms. Patients with lymphatic malformations or lymphedema may develop lymphangitis, presenting with fever, chills, achiness, and headache. Characteristics of lymphangitis include a red "streak" following the course of the infected lymphatic channels as well as enlarged, tender lymph nodes in the area of lymphatic drainage. Skin infection or local trauma often precedes the symptoms (Figure 20).

Lymphedema

Swelling from blocked lymphatic vessels or lymph node problems.

Dysplasia

Abnormally formed.

Lymphangitis

Inflammation of lymphatic channels due to infection/inflammation.

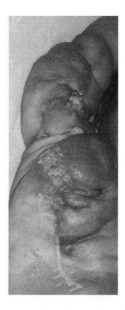

Figure 20   Lymphatic malformation with cellulitis.

Prompt evaluation and treatment with antibiotics is necessary.

75. What are some of the major types of lymphatic malformations?

Other names for lymphatic malformations are cystic hygromas or lymphangiomas. Sometimes lymphatic malformations have small blebs (sacs) on the surface of the skin. These may bleed or drain clear or pink/red fluid. Laser therapy to seal these blebs may help prevent the leakage. Thin sanitary napkins placed on clothing may also absorb the drainage and prevent embarrassing leakage. Cystic hygromas are larger lymphatic malformations, fluid-filled sacs, caused by the failure of normal lymphatic development in the neck region. Cystic hygromas can be associated with some syndromes and chromosomal abnormalities.

Lymphangiectasia

Abnormal dilation of lymphatic vessels.

Lymphangiectasia is a term for lymphatic vessels that are abnormally dilated. This condition often occurs in the abdomen, and collections of fluid, called *ascites*, may occur. The abdomen will appear distended, and treatment will be required. When lymphangiectasia occurs, therapy is challenging. Lymphatic fluid containing proteins and lymphocytes may collect in the abdomen or other areas, often requiring drainage via a catheter and replacement with intravenous gamma-globulin and/or albumin.

Lymphangioma circumscriptum refers to discrete patches of microcysts (small sacs of lymphatic fluid) that appear as a clear or colored (red, brown, pink) and sometimes thickened area on the skin with protuberant blebs (small cysts), which may ooze serosanguinous (clear or pink) fluid. They may occur on any area of the skin and sometimes on the tongue or mucous membranes of the mouth. They often become more pronounced in the peripubertal years.

76. What is lymphedema?

For more information on lymphedema see 100 Questions & Answers About Lymphedema by Thiadens, Stewart, and Stout (availabe online at www.jblearning.com).

Lymphedema is a term for swelling that occurs when protein-rich lymphatic fluid collects outside of the lymphatic vessels (Figure 21). It is a type of fluid retention that is caused when lymphatic fluid is unable to circulate properly within the lymphatic system due to missing or damaged lymphatic vessels and/or nodes. The limbs become engorged (swollen) with fluid. Left untreated, the extremities become indurated (firm) due to lack of mobilization of the excess fluid. Skin changes may also ensue.

There are two main types of lymphedema: primary and secondary.

- *Primary lymphedema* (or inherited lymphedema) occurs when a person's lymphatic system develops abnormally. Even though a person may be born with this condition, symptoms may not appear until puberty (lymphedema praecox) or later in life (lymphedema tarda). One rare type of primary (congenital) lymphedema of infancy is Milroy disease. Lymphedema may also be present in association with genetic syndromes such as Turner syndrome and others as noted in Table 9.
- *Secondary lymphedema* is more common and often results from damage to the lymphatic system from another cause, such as surgery, radiation therapy, trauma, or certain infections, especially filariasis, a tropical disease caused by a parasite. Many women who have had breast cancer surgery have secondary lymphedema of their arms.

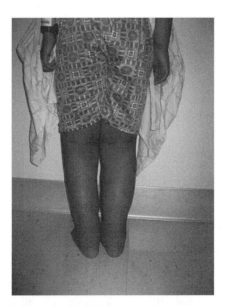

Figure 21   Lymphedema.

Table 9   Lymphatic Malformation Syndromes

Name of Syndrome	Clinical Features
Gorham syndrome (Gorham-Stout syndrome) Disappearing bone disease	Lymphangiomatosis associated with bony destruction
Milroy disease	Lymphedema present at birth
Meige syndrome Lymphedema praecox	Lymphedema appears later in life
Hennekam syndrome	Lymphedema of face, genitals, limbs; characteristic skeletal and facial abnormalities
Yellow nail syndrome	Discolored thick nails, lung problems, and lymphedema
Intestinal lymphangiectasia	Dilation of intestinal lymphatics causing loss of lymph fluid into the gastrointestinal tract, hypoproteinemia (low serum protein levels), edema, and lymphocytopenia (low lymphocyte count)
Lymphedema with distichiasis	Lymphedema, extra row of eyelashes (distichiasis), other related problems including abnormal spinal canal
Turner syndrome or Noonan syndrome	May have lymphatic malformations and/or lymphedema

Lymphedema can be challenging to treat and manage. It can be disfiguring and have psychological implications.

Lymphedema can be challenging to treat and manage. It can be disfiguring and have psychological implications. Lymphedema most often affects a person's arm(s) and/or leg(s). It can progress from a latency stage (not yet evident or active) to reversible lymphedema (which improves with elevation of the extremity). Symptoms may include swelling, pain, weakness, a feeling of tightness, less flexibility, or heaviness in an affected area such as arms or legs. A later stage is spontaneously irreversible lymphedema, where there is fibrosis (thickening of the tissue) followed by *elephantiasis* (firm tissue with skin changes). It is nearly impossible to correct this severe form of lymphedema by conservative means, and surgery may be the only alternative.

There are different approaches to the treatment of lymphedema. Your doctor can help you find an approach that is right for you, such as:

- Symptom management
- Bandaging, compression stocking or sleeve
- Compression devices
- Exercise
- Massage
- Medication
- Liposuction
- Surgery

There are many helpful resources on the Internet for patients with lymphedema.

- The National Lymphedema Network
- MayoClinic.com (Search for "lymphedema.")
- Lymphedema People

77. I've heard of lymphatic drainage massage therapy. Do you recommend it?

Complete decongestive lymphatic drainage therapy (CDT) consists of several components: (1) manual lymph drainage (MLD), which entails precise manual massage along the lymphatic system to clear and decompress the abnormal lymphatic vessels at the site of lymphedema; (2) bandaging or wrapping of the area after MLD to prevent refilling of lymphatic fluid; (3) proper skin care and diet; (4) compression garments; and (5) exercises.

Complete decongestive lymphatic drainage therapy (CDT)

Form of physical therapy for lymphedema that involves massage therapy to mobilize lymphatic fluid, followed by wrapping the affected area.

This therapy is available at certified centers where physical therapists have undergone specific training in this technique. Parents of young children should approach this therapy very cautiously. Many therapists are uncomfortable performing lymphatic drainage massage on most pediatric patients.

The National Lymphedema Network (www.lymphnet. org) offers updated guidelines on their Web site, and other professional lymphology associations such as the International Lymphology Association have useful information online.

78. What precautions should I be aware of regarding lymphatic malformations?

People who have a lymphatic malformation are at greater risk for infection. They should practice proper oral and skin hygiene to help prevent infection. Sometimes antibiotics are prescribed to prevent infection, especially when lymphatic malformations are in the area of the mouth, which normally harbors bacteria that can enter facial lymphatic malformations. Patients who have large lymphatic abnormalities of the abdomen or chest, which impair the normal lymphatic flow, may require a special low-fat diet. In severe cases, fluid may need to be drained from these lesions.

People affected with lymphedema are at a greater risk for infection due to the impaired circulation of lymphatic fluid. They should take care to avoid situations that might cause infection; even simple scratches or cuts to the skin or insect bites can cause infection, or *lymphangitis* (see Question 74), in people with lymphedema. Thus, patients with lymphedema should maintain excellent skin hygiene (especially in the affected area), and patients with lymphatic abnormalities of the lower extremities should always wear firm-soled shoes or slippers and should not walk barefoot. Patients with lymphedema of the upper extremity should avoid blood pressure measurements and venipuncture (blood drawing), injections, and intravenous insertion in the affected extremity. Patients should seek medical attention for new onset of pain, redness, or swelling.

Patients who have lymphedema or complex lymphatic malformations can obtain, at no cost, a Lymphedema Alertband (www.lymphedema.com/alertband.htm). Air travel may be challenging for patients with lymphedema, and compression garments, prevention of dehydration, and elevation of the affected extremity are warranted. The National Lymphedema Network provides updated guidelines regarding air travel for patients with lymphedema which can be found online (www.lymphnet. org—search for "air travel").

79. Why are compression devices recommended, and how do they work?

In order to mobilize the buildup of excess fluid in the tissues, compression devices are sometimes recommended. These devices provide pumping action, forcing the fluids to be absorbed by the circulatory system. There are many types of lymphatic compression devices. Some pumps have been found to exert excess pressure and damage the superficial lymphatics. With *intermittent pneumatic compression devices*, an inflatable garment covering the affected extremity is connected to a pneumatic pump that intermittently fills and deflates the garment, massaging and increasing lymphatic drainage. These devices are generally used at night. They are considered durable medical equipment and may require prior authorization from your insurance company. It is best to work with a lymphatic specialist who can guide you in choosing the best pump as well as justify the medical necessity for the device, facilitating insurance coverage.

Elastic compression stockings or sleeves may benefit patients with venous or lymphatic issues by providing additional support to veins and lymphatic vessels if veins and valves have become weakened over time. Compression sleeves and stockings come in a variety of colors, materials, and compression classes. Although light compression stockings can be purchased over the counter or online, it is best to check with your doctor to get a professional recommendation about the type of sleeve of stocking that is right for you or your child. The physician can write a prescription and refer you to a store or pharmacy in your area with a qualified fitter on staff. Plan to replace regularly worn compression devices every 6 to 9 months as the elastic becomes worn and less supportive. During pregnancy, women with vascular and lymphatic malformations may benefit from using compression sleeves or stockings.

80. When is sclerotherapy used to treat lymphatic malformations, how does it work, and what are the complications?

Large sacs such as those seen in lymphatic malformations contain fluid. This fluid can be removed and replaced with a substance that causes inflammation within the sac, which ultimately sticks together, closing off the sac. This is the principle of sclerotherapy. Several medications have been used for sclerotherapy, including bleomycin, doxycycline, and picibanil (OK-432). Bleomycin is a form of chemotherapy; however, when used as a sclerotherapy agent, it is administered into the sac at a very low dose. Although most patients tolerate bleomycin treatment without major issues, patients receiving bleomycin should be monitored for pulmonary (lung) toxicity prior to and once they have received this agent. Doxycycline is a type of antibiotic. Picibanil is an investigational drug; it is contraindicated in patients with penicillin allergy because it is prepared in the presence of penicillin.

81. What are some of the syndromes associated with lymphatic malformations?

Lymphatic abnormalities may be isolated, with lymphatic cysts or lymphedema in one location in the body, or they may be multifocal, occurring in adjacent or distant areas in the body. Many, but not all lymphatic syndromes also involve developmental delay, with abnormal facial and skeletal features and/or abnormally developed organs such as the kidneys. Lymphatic abnormalities may occur in conjunction with other vascular anomalies, such as Klippel-Trenaunay syndrome. Table 9 lists some syndromes that may have lymphatic malformations and/or lymphedema as a dominant feature (see Question 76). This list is by no means exhaustive.

Inherited disorders with lymphatic abnormalities can be transmitted either as **autosomal** recessive or dominant traits. One abnormal gene inherited from each parent is necessary in an autosomal recessively transmitted disorder such as Hennekam syndrome; only one gene from one parent is necessary for expression of an

Autosomal

Inherited on non-sex chromosomes.

autosomal dominantly transmitted disorder such as Noonan syndrome. Sporadic mutations can always occur in diseases. In such cases, even though a mutation may be genetic, it is not inherited from either parent. Instead, the genetic mutation occurs spontaneously, or at random, in the patient.

Patients with Gorham syndrome (Gorham-Stout syndrome), also known as disappearing bone disease, experience **osteolysis**, generally due to lymphatic malformations. This disorder can lead to severe misshapen bones, pain, and functional limitations. Treatment thus far is based on symptoms as they occur, often requiring surgery.

Osteolysis

Bony destruction.

Congenital lymphedema, presenting at birth, is known as Milroy disease. Lymphedema praecox, also known as Meige syndrome (Nonne-Milroy-Meige syndrome), presents in the second to fifth decades of life, often in the peripubertal years, and generally affects the legs. Evaluation by lymphoscintigram, (a procedure which traces the transit time of a radioactive marker that is taken up by the lymphatics) often shows abnormalities in the caliber of the affected lymphatic vessels.

Hennekam syndrome is a rare, multifocal lymphedema condition affecting the face, lungs, intestines, genitals, and limbs, with characteristic skeletal and facial features such as a flat face, depressed and wide nasal bridge, down-slanting opening between the eyelids, widely spaced eyes, and low-set ears.

Patients with yellow nail syndrome (also known as primary lymphedema associated with yellow nails and pleural effusion) experience discolored thick nails, respiratory problems, sinus infections, and lymphedema.

Intestinal lymphangiectasia (IL) +/− protein-losing enteropathy (PLE) represent conditions characterized by the dilation (IL) or obstruction (PLE) of intestinal lymphatics, causing loss of lymph fluid and proteins into the gastrointestinal tract, leading to hypoproteinemia (low serum protein levels), **edema**, and lymphocytopenia (low lymphocyte count). In addition to supportive care to maintain protein levels (e.g., albumin and/or intravenous immunoglobulin infusions), patients with these disorders often benefit from special high-protein, low-fat diets, with medium chain triglyceride (MCT) supplementation, which is available as formula or oil. In these cases, working with a knowledgeable registered dietician or **nutritionist** who is an expert in dietary care is optimal. A Web site with excellent information and resources is www.littleleakers.com.

Lymphedema with distichiasis involves lymphedema of the extremities, an extra row of eyelashes (distichiasis), and other related problems including spinal canal abnormalities. A FOXC2 mutation has been identified in patients having this rare disorder.

Patients with Turner syndrome or Noonan syndrome may have lymphatic malformations and/or lymphedema along with numerous skeletal, facial, genitourinary, and cardiovascular anomalies. Noonan syndrome, which affects males and females, is characterized by a webbed neck, congenital heart defects, lymphedema, short stature, learning difficulties, pectus excavatum (midline indentation of chest), blood clotting disorders, and characteristic facial features. Turner syndrome has similar features and affects females only.

Lymphangioleiomyomatosis (LAM) affects the lung and is characterized by abnormal smooth muscle cell and lymphatic proliferation leading to pulmonary

Edema
Swelling.

Nutritionist
Expert in dietary care.

Lymphatic Malformations

cysts, lymphatic fluid collections (chylous pleural effusion), and respiratory symptoms. This disorder, which primarily affects women of childbearing age or (rarely) patients with tuberous sclerosis, is not discussed in detail in this book, however further information regarding LAM is available online through MedlinePlus (MedlinePlus.gov) and the National Heart, Lung, and Blood Institute (www.nhlbi.nih.gov) by searching for the term "LAM." Details regarding research studies for patients affected by LAM may be found through the National Heart, Lung, and Blood Institute.

Table 9, Lymphatic Malformation Syndromes, provides more information regarding the syndromes associated with lymphatic malformations (see Question 76).

PART FIVE

Living with Vascular Anomalies

Everywhere we go people stare and make comments. What can we say?

Should an adult or child avoid certain sports or activities?

What are the long-term health implications for me or my child?

More . . .

82. Where we live there are no specialists familiar with complicated vascular lesions. What should we do?

It is always worth seeking expert opinions from physicians who see many patients with these disorders. If you live in an area without easy access to a physician specialist or a vascular anomalies center, consider researching through a patient support organization for referrals to specialists. You may even be able to arrange a brief, preliminary phone or email conference with a specialist before scheduling an appointment. Because this area of specialty is often not well understood by general pediatricians or internists, it is important to have your care and treatment overseen by a vascular anomalies specialist. These physicians can work with you or your child's primary care physician to ensure that proper monitoring can be ongoing.

It is always worth seeking expert opinions from physicians who see many patients with these disorders.

Many families find themselves traveling long distances to specialists in order to be treated by someone with considerable experience treating a high volume of patients with vascular lesions. For many patients this means seeing a physician who is considered "out of network" by their insurance plan. Depending on your insurance, you may need to get a referral to a specialist or you may need to clarify what your insurance covers as out of network benefits. You may be able to get a letter from your primary care doctor explaining that this care is medically necessary and not available through your regular physician network. Although managing insurance hassles is never pleasant, having your care managed by an expert specialist will ensure the best outcome and will be well worth these inconveniences.

83. Insurance does not cover procedures that are recommended for our child. What can we do?

Navigating through the maze of health insurance is a common challenge for families affected by vascular anomalies. Parents may learn after the fact that certain necessary procedures are not covered. Insurance companies may deny coverage initially for procedures they consider to be elective or cosmetic, such as various types of reconstructive or plastic surgery, necessary dental work, or even procedures to treat obvious medical needs.

During annual insurance election periods, some families "shop around" to determine what insurance plan provides the best coverage based on their individual needs. Families with two insured parents may research which parent's plan best suits the medical needs of their child. You may also choose to investigate what other resources may be available to you or your child, such as through government services and/or foundations dedicated to serving children with special needs. A social worker or patient advocate at your hospital or vascular anomalies center may be able to help you get started. Working with a dedicated case worker from the insurance plan can expedite the often arduous process.

Every patient's needs are different, but during a time of active treatment, families may need to make frequent trips to their doctor and specialist, requiring more comprehensive insurance coverage. Later, during a period of maintenance, families may only need occasional medical appointments to monitor the child's vascular anomaly intermittently.

Most importantly, try to stay calm and polite with the various insurance representatives with whom you interact no matter how frustrating this can be. Be sure to take detailed notes, noting the day, time, representative's name, and a summary of your conversation. Keep carefully documented notes and correspondence from the various physicians and specialists you see, including laboratory and radiologic studies. Keep photographs and a journal of significant medical and developmental events. In the event that your insurance company denies a claim, your documentation and supporting letters from physicians will make your case for appeal much stronger. If your insurance company denies your appeal, you may file a formal appeal or grievance and even contact your State Board of Insurance.

Consider contacting one of the disease-specific support groups for tips on how to navigate insurance coverage for you or your child (see the Appendix). You may find it helpful to talk with a fellow parent or a parent advocate who has faced a similar challenge. Many times, though, families find that determination, letters describing medical necessity from a physician specialist, thorough documentation, and considerable patience can result in the desired coverage outcome. Physicians are accustomed to this request and are generally willing to help you in this process.

Many families find their health insurance does not make it easy for them to get their claims covered. Even when a physician does not accept your insurance plan or there is much red tape, there are several important resources to help you work through these obstacles. Insurance coverage for certain procedures (e.g., laser treatments) can vary by state. The National Organization for Vascular Anomalies (NOVA) offers a brochure which can be found at the NOVA Web site (www.novanews.org), "Health Insurance Coverage for Vascular Anomalies: How to Appeal a Denial of Benefits;" the Vascular Birthmarks Foundation (www.birthmark.org) provides a document, "How to Appeal an Insurance Denial or Request Out-of-Network Treatment," to help walk you through the process; and the Sturge-Weber Foundation's "Position Paper on the Necessity for the Treatment of Port Wine Stains" offers medical references to support your appeal which you can find at the foundation's Web site (www.sturge-weber.org).

The Kaiser Family Foundation Web site (www.kff.org) provides factual health policy information regarding Medicaid, Medicare, and prescription drugs. The National Association of Insurance Commissioners (www.naic.org) provides state-by-state information regarding health-care insurance.

Additionally, you or your child may be eligible for disability (Supplemental Security Income [SSI]) benefits if certain eligibility requirements are fulfilled. Details are available at Social Security Online (www.ssa.gov).

84. Everywhere we go people stare and make comments. What can we say?

Anything you want! Constantly fielding questions, rude comments, and stares from strangers is one of the most difficult challenges faced by children and adults with vascular anomalies. Many families find it exhausting to respond to stares and comments from the public everywhere they go. While you or your child may be known and understood among your circle of family and friends, the larger public will always have questions. One adult with very prominent facial vascular anomalies has commented that once people get to know him, they don't notice his facial differences. You may find this to be true, too.

Many parents of young children affected by hemangiomas, lymphatic malformations, port wine stains, Sturge-Weber syndrome, or other vascular anomalies that cause facial differences feel that how they respond in public is very important for their children. Even at an early age, children and their siblings learn powerful lessons and coping strategies by observing how their parents navigate questions, comments, and stares from strangers. Try to develop a few rehearsed responses that you can draw on. You may want to brainstorm and network with other parents through a parent-support network to find out what strategies worked best for them. As hard as it is, remember that you are modeling skills for your child and setting an example for him or her. Your confident, clear response sends a message to strangers, and more importantly to your child and his or her siblings, that your child is beautiful, loved, and someone of whom you are very proud.

It is important to remember that very often stares or questions from strangers or young children are a reaction due to surprise or lack of awareness. You may choose to respond to inquiries with simple educational responses, or you may decide to have a preprinted information card handy to present basic facts about your or your child's vascular anomaly. These questions can be valuable opportunities to educate others about vascular anomalies. The Sturge-Weber Foundation has "Check It Out" cards that a family can hand out when they don't wish to answer questions, but still want to create awareness and educate the public about port wine stains, Sturge-Weber syndrome, and Klippel-Trenaunay syndrome.

Your confident, clear response sends a message to strangers, and more importantly to your child and his or her siblings, that your child is beautiful, loved, and someone of whom you are very proud.

Each card offers a brief explanation and details for how to learn more.

Everyone has their own strategy about how to respond to comments, ranging from dispassionate explanations to surprising snappy quips. Some ideas are:

- "My child has a medical condition that is caused by blood vessels that formed abnormally."
- "She has a vascular abnormality that is called a hemangioma. I can spell it for you . . . H-E-M-A-N-G-I-O-M-A."
- "I noticed you admiring my son. He is a beautiful baby, isn't he?"

Whatever approach you choose, it is wise to prepare yourself and an affected child for these encounters. One thing is certain, there will be questions.

Jessica says:

Luckily our son's hemangioma was not in a conspicuous area—it was hidden by his diaper so we didn't have much explaining to do. But once I was changing him in a public restroom and an elderly lady wanted to help me. I accepted her help without thought, but just before I opened his diaper, I remembered the hemangioma. I stopped and said to the woman, "Oh, just so you're not alarmed, he has a large tumor on his tush." Then I opened the diaper. She made no comments and had no reaction. She continued to play with him while I changed the diaper. It was no big deal to her, but without my "warning," she may have been taken aback.

85. What support is available to families?

There may be a vascular anomaly support group of patients/families in your community. You can ask your physician to provide you with names of families who have agreed to share their experience with newly diagnosed patients, as they can help you to see the "light at the end of the tunnel" or at least feel less alone. The Appendix lists various patient support organizations that have support groups or may be able to connect you to other families with similar experiences. Many of the support organizations have online communities, message boards, blogs, or "chat" areas.

You may also find help through other more general organizations by looking online for support groups related to caregiving, facial differences, rare diseases, parents with children who have disabilities, or children with special needs. Depending on where you live, you may find support groups that meet in person close to where you live. Many families also find support through community and church organizations.

Don't be afraid, too, to reach out to friends, neighbors, and family. You may be surprised to find so many people rallying for you and your family; often people want to help but they don't want to "intrude." Consider making very specific requests of what you need help with—is it yard work, picking up other children from school, house cleaning, shopping for groceries, babysitting? Even help with small daily tasks can be a big relief. Consider other types of requests also that may make life easier. Maybe you'd like to meet a friend for coffee just to talk. Or maybe you could use some help creating a Web site to notify friends and family about updates.

86. Should my child's condition affect my parenting?

Many parents of children with medical issues struggle with parenting issues during their child's illness and treatment.

As tempting as it might be to overlook certain behavioral challenges during treatment, it is very important to be consistent with your children and to set limits that are age appropriate based on your child's developmental stage. Believe it or not, children actually are comforted by routines and consistency. It is important, too, that, as much as possible, your child's experience (and that of his or her siblings) should be "normalized." You may find it helpful to look at popular parenting books online, at a local library, or bookstore for parenting tips and support. The Sturge-Weber Foundation has a comprehensive resource guide that discusses all aspects of raising a child with a port wine birthmark and Sturge-Weber syndrome.

Finally, consider seeking professional help if you need it. For some people talking to a professional therapist or counselor can be enormously helpful. Talking with a therapist may help you to see your own situation more objectively and to focus on positive aspects of your family and the medical experience. If you are considering seeing a therapist, ask around for recommendations from others. Finding the person who is right for you can make all the difference.

87. Do you have suggestions for how to balance the needs of our other children?

This is a very common question from parents. The other children may have confusing feelings and unexpected behavioral changes. For example:

- Siblings may feel left out or neglected by other family members.
- They may feel responsible or worry that they caused the vascular anomaly.

Living with Vascular Anomalies

- They may worry that the vascular lesion is contagious and that they might be affected.
- They may worry that their brother or sister may die.
- They may be embarrassed by the unwanted public attention this medical condition brings your family.
- They may begin to act out in a way that calls attention to their own minor ailments as attention-seeking behavior.
- Often siblings become protective of children with medical conditions, including vascular anomalies.

The best way to understand the needs of your other children is to talk with them honestly and directly in a way that makes sense based on their age and development.

The best way to understand the needs of your other children is to talk with them honestly and directly in a way that makes sense based on their age and development. Some parents choose to ask open-ended questions of their other children to encourage discussion, such as, "What do you think about your sister's hemangioma?" Many parents try to respond to a young child's questions or concerns with honest answers that are age appropriate but not overly detailed.

You may want to rehearse your explanations or conversation in advance, or you may want to get suggestions or advice from other parents who have been through this themselves. If your care is coordinated through a large medical center, you might get suggestions from professionals on the treatment team such as child life specialists, social workers, or child psychologists.

Some parents try to find ways to involve their other children in the medical process to help them understand what is happening and to help them feel included. Possible activities might include having a young child help select supplies at the drug store or help with caregiving activities for his or her sibling.

During your child's treatment, it is important to spend time with your other children so they do not feel neglected. Some couples take turns spending time with their other children. In some families, extended family members such as grandparents, aunts, and uncles as well as close family friends can schedule time to do something special with the other children.

88. Is it common for parents to be depressed?

Yes, depression is very common. In addition to postpartum depression, there are many overwhelming feelings that emerge when a newborn has a vascular anomaly. Parents may experience any range of emotions including anger, guilt, fear, worry, depression, isolation, and grief. It is very hard for parents who have waited hopefully and expectantly for their new baby to suddenly learn at birth or shortly after that their baby has a vascular anomaly. New parents can feel upset that this diagnosis was not determined before birth, especially when all prenatal testing results were fine. Mothers may feel upset because they "did everything right" during their pregnancy. All of these feelings are completely normal and very common.

Parents also experience stressful feelings when there is uncertainty about the diagnosis or prognosis of a child's condition. It can be frustrating to wait on diagnostic tests and expert opinions and even more frustrating when a diagnosis is not easily confirmed. Many parents become angry, overwhelmed, and fearful because they feel helpless about being able to resolve their child's condition. Sometimes these feelings derive from uncertainty about the future and/or confusion as to the diagnosis. A period of recommended "watchful waiting" without any intervention can also make parents anxious and concerned about whether enough is being done.

You may find that some of the anxious feelings you have can be relieved by being honest with yourself about your feelings, by seeking professional or community support for yourself, and by being well informed. Make certain that you ask any questions that are on your mind and that you understand what the physicians have communicated to you at the end of each visit. It is very helpful to write down questions as you think of them and bring this list to office visits. You may also want to take notes during your doctor's visits or ask a friend or relative to come along to do this for you. Most of all, remember that what you are feeling is normal.

Jeannine says:

My husband and I were terribly distraught upon learning of our daughter's vascular anomaly and subsequent PHACES diagnosis. We had tried 8 years to have her and were thrilled to finally be pregnant. All prenatal testing indicated that she was healthy. So we were shocked, devastated, and overwhelmed upon learning otherwise. There were days that it was almost more than we could bear, but as all of her tests were completed and we educated ourselves on her condition, we felt more in control. Leaning on our friends and family was instrumental in getting us through, especially during those early days. They lifted our spirits. We also went for individual and family counseling, which was invaluable to us. In our counseling sessions, we learned to tolerate each other's coping styles and were able to keep our family intact and thrive through it all. We were able to lean on our therapist instead of each other during those times when neither one of us had the strength to help the other. Going for counseling was one of the best choices we made for ourselves during this time when all our energies were spent taking care of our daughter and getting her through. We needed to get to a place where we were strong so that we could care for our daughter.

89. What studies, clinical trials, or registries are there?

This is an exciting time for research in vascular anomalies, as more laboratories are publishing relevant manuscripts. The genetics and possible mechanisms of action are being worked out, and new medications are being discovered. Your physician can discuss current registries and clinical trials. We anticipate further milestones in diagnosis and treatment.

Professional meetings focusing on vascular anomalies serve as a forum for interested physicians to share their research results and scientific/clinical observations. Physicians and scientists also discuss challenging cases, learn from each other, and sometimes design studies. It is best to inquire at multidisciplinary vascular anomalies centers if there are any clinical trials seeking patients to see if you or your child is eligible to participate.

90. Should an adult or child avoid certain sports or activities?

Sports, exercise, and physical activity are important for good health. Physical activity improves circulation and may even help with symptom management in some patients with vascular anomalies. It is very important, though, to protect an affected area from trauma or blows to the body that might occur in certain sports such as handball, soccer, volleyball, and dodgeball. An affected area could possibly be made worse or bleed (even internally) in extreme situations.

Generally, activities such as swimming, tennis, running, walking, golf, and biking are best. Check with your doctor for suggestions about activities or precautions/safety equipment to help you or your child stay active.

91. Is there a prenatal test for vascular anomalies?

Vascular malformations, RICH-type hemangiomas, and some liver hemangiomas may be detected via prenatal ultrasound. When a genetic mutation has been previously identified in the family, an amniocentesis or **chorionic villus sampling** test can be performed to study if the mutation is present in the fetus. Alternatively, by using in vitro fertilization (IVF), pre-implantation genetic testing can be performed on fertilized eggs prior to implantation to select for an unaffected offspring. Pre-implantation genetic testing can only be used if a known gene defect has been identified.

Chorionic villus sampling

Prenatal test used to determine chromosome abnormality or genetic defect in the fetus.

92. Is there anything I did to cause this?

No. Most often a vascular malformation occurs during embryonic development as the result of a small, focal mistake during the process of rapid cell division as the embryo develops. Although vascular anomalies may be influenced by hormonal changes and genetics (which are completely beyond an individual's control), anomalies usually occur sporadically.

There are many cultural beliefs and stories that have been passed along for centuries implying that the vascular anomaly was caused because during pregnancy the woman thought something she shouldn't have, saw something unpleasant, or ate red fruits such as strawberries, raspberries, or cherries. This is simply *not true*.

Certainly good health habits, exercise, and proper nutrition are very important during pregnancy, but there is nothing new parents have done to cause a vascular anomaly.

Certainly good health habits, exercise, and proper nutrition are very important during pregnancy, but there is nothing new parents have done to cause a vascular anomaly. While some vascular anomalies are genetic and run in families, the vast majority are sporadic, with no known cause.

Susan and Ken say:

Every parent wonders if there is anything he or she could or should have done differently so that their child would not have had a vascular anomaly. We certainly did. Our doctors assured us that there was nothing we could have done differently, and that it wasn't our fault. In particular, women may feel more responsible, because you are carrying the baby for 9 months and feel that you have some control over the development of the child and thus hemangiomas. Seeing our newborn with facial hemangiomas is a difficult thing to live with, and it is emotionally challenging. This was especially the case because our older child was not born with hemangiomas and we had not seen or heard of them before our second child was born. The good news is that it is much more difficult for the parents than the children. Our daughter was not in any pain or discomfort and was too young to have any negative feelings about the way she looked. The better news is that there are effective treatment options available, and the prognosis is very hopeful. The early months are by far the most challenging, and it gets better after that.

Johanna says:

"Do not blame yourself," I remember our specialist telling me. My husband and I were just overwhelmed and had a million questions. I thought I had done something wrong—eaten the wrong thing . . . all of these thoughts raced through my head. But as the doctor explained there was nothing I had done wrong. The blame was something I learned to do away with as I became more informed through research and the doctor's guidance. The doctor's support and explanations were very useful. It made me understand and accept how much more important it was to treat my daughter than to look for blame.

93. The number of physicians and tests is overwhelming. How can I keep everything straight? How do I manage taking off from work for all of my child's necessary appointments?

Keeping a separate loose-leaf notebook with tabbed sections to insert business cards of all healthcare providers, a calendar for appointments, tests, and medication schedules, and other information will prove very helpful. Also request copies of all laboratory, radiology, and surgical reports, collect correspondences among physicians, and keep a list of ongoing questions. Request copies of all radiologic studies, preferably on CDs, and bring these as well as all medications to the visits with physicians. Keeping detailed records will assist in insurance claims, answering your doctor's questions, and recording information that could easily be forgotten over time.

Some suggested sections for a notebook follow:

- Section for business cards of physicians and ancillary healthcare providers
- Calendar to list all physician visits (name, subspecialty)
- Test results: blood, radiologic, and other tests
- Consultation letters and medical reports
- Patient information printouts from Web sites
- Questions for healthcare providers
- Medications and dosage amounts
- Pharmacy information
- Insurance card information (copy both sides)
- Documentation of claims and communication with your insurance company

Often families of two working parents struggle trying to balance the needs of their child and their workplace. It can seem as if physician and specialist appointments are always in conflict with the work schedule. Many parents try to find ways to minimize their absences from work. When possible, try to schedule early morning or late afternoon appointments with physicians and check to see if some tests, such as MRI scans, are available on weekends. Some doctors may see patients in evenings and/or on weekends. Check if there is any flexibility in your work schedule to accommodate these appointments. Depending on your child's needs, you may explore options available from your workplace through Family Medical Leave Act (FMLA) legislation. To learn about the different types of FMLA leave, including continuous, intermittent, and reduced-schedule FMLA leave, look online for more detailed guidelines through the U.S. Department of Labor at www.dol.gov and search for the term "FMLA."

94. How do you recommend discussing complicated medical and psychosocial issues with young children?

You know your child better than anyone. Try to find books with characters or themes that appeal to your child. There are more and more books written to explain complicated medical and psychosocial issues in a child-friendly way; some of these are listed in Table 10. Siblings will also benefit from these resources.

Try to be prepared to answer any questions your child might have. If you get stuck, many vascular anomalies centers have social workers, child life specialists, and psychologists on staff that are there to help. Although young children do not need to be overwhelmed with medical information, explaining things to them simply and directly can go a long way. Being informed about procedures, tests, and exams will help reduce a child's anxiety and fear.

Table 10 Recommended Books for Young Children

Title/author	Description
Buddy Booby's Birthmark Donna and Evan Ducker	Based on his experience growing up with a port wine stain birthmark, child-author Evan Ducker gives young readers a hero who loves the thing that makes him different from others. This story's message about the importance of tolerance and self-acceptance resonates with children who have birthmarks themselves.
Dandelion Don Freeman	The story of a lion who is turned away from a party because he is so overdressed that his friends can't recognize him. Young children will enjoy this funny story and the underlying message that it's always best to be yourself.
Freckleface Strawberry Julianne Moore	How to accept yourself the way you are, via a story about a girl with freckles.
I Love You Because You're You Liza Baker	Liza Baker's rhyming picture book is told from the point of view of a mother fox to her fox child. This short and simple story underscores the mother's unconditional love for her child.
I'm Gonna Like Me: Letting Off a Little Self-Esteem Jamie Lee Curtis	Jamie Lee Curtis is bound to entertain young children with the upbeat, positive rhyming message and the funny illustrations with detailed visual puns. Curtis underscores the importance of liking oneself even when mistakes are made, such as putting out a birthday cake with a fire extinguisher!
The Legend of Spookley the Square Pumpkin Joe Troiano	Because Spookley is a square pumpkin, he is teased by his friends and other round pumpkins who don't appreciate his difference. Readers will enjoy the plot twist in Troiano's story when a Halloween windstorm challenges everyone in the pumpkin patch except Spookley. Spookley fans may also enjoy the DVD version of the story.
Mookey the Monkey Gets Over Being Teased Heather Lonczak	This story is about a monkey who is teased because he was born with no hair and looks very different from his friends. This book provides a great way for parents or teachers to start a conversation about teasing and bullying and to talk about strategies for responding to teasing.

Table 10   Recommended Books for Young Children (*Continued*)

Title/author	Description
The Okay Book and *It's Okay to Be Different* Todd Parr	Young children will enjoy the brightly colored silly illustrations in both of these books by Todd Parr. Parr balances the silly and the serious, always encouraging young readers with the message to celebrate what makes them unique.
Happy Birthday to You! and *Oh, the Places You'll Go!* Dr. Seuss	These classic Dr. Seuss titles have fanciful illustrations, funny rhymes, and powerful messages of resilience. Children young and old will enjoy reading these stories together.
Little Tree: A Story for Children with Serious Medical Problems Joyce C. Mills, PhD	This story is a helpful way of discussing a serious medical illness in a child-friendly way.
What About Me? When Brothers and Sisters Get Sick Allan Peterkin, MD	This story addresses the unique needs of siblings who often feel left out during the treatment process.

Jeannine says:

As our child got older, she became more and more aware of what was happening to her and started to get anxious before her surgeries and yearly tests. I didn't think that a 2-year-old would really know what was going on, but I was so wrong! Because we flew to New York for treatment, her anxiety would start as soon as we touched down in New York. The then 2-year-old said, "Mom, plane, car, home, now!" It broke my heart, but what we were doing for her was absolutely necessary, so I decided that from that moment on I would tell her what we were going to be doing so that she would be prepared and there would be no surprises for her, hoping this would alleviate some of her anxiety. So, when she was about 3.5 years old and having yet another surgery and battery of tests, I sat her down before our trip and simply explained that we were going to New York for her checkup (just like the Callou TV character does) and that she was going to see all of her doctors. She asked me why, and I told her, "The doctor has to fix your nose, remember?" She hesitated for a moment and I watched her as she took in all that I said. She simply replied, "OK, Mom, I can do it, but will you hold my hand?" Of course, I held her hand, and the trip went better than most of the ones before. She was really calm at the hospital—no crying this time—and was so cooperative with all the hospital staff. Everyone around me thought it was crazy of me to explain it to her, but I was right—it was the best thing I could have done for her at that time.

95. My child's doctor mentioned that a tracheotomy may be necessary. What is this?

A **tracheotomy** is a procedure to insert a breathing tube into the airway. Usually an otolaryngologist—also know as an ear, nose, and throat (ENT) doctor—performs the procedure. Situations where this procedure may be necessary include a large hemangioma of the airway or compression of the airway due to a large venous or lymphatic malformation. A tracheotomy is not usually the first choice of treatment; however, a tracheotomy may be inserted in an emergency situation or prophylactically if there is concern about progression or swelling. Sometimes a tracheotomy is temporarily inserted preoperatively if the surgeons are concerned that **debulking** surgery or embolization/sclerotherapy will cause swelling. This type of tracheotomy can be removed once postoperative swelling has subsided.

Tracheotomy
Procedure to create an airway opening in the event the airway is obstructed, either internally (e.g., by a hemangioma) or externally (from swelling or a mass pressing on the airway).

Debulking
Surgical removal or reduction of the mass of a vascular growth.

96. The medication prescribed for my child is not approved by the FDA for this disorder. Should I be worried? What about generic drugs—are they okay?

According to a 2008 report in the *New England Journal of Medicine*, "Off-label prescribing—the prescription of a medication in a manner different from that approved by the FDA—is legal and common" and is best practiced when there are supporting data in the literature for use of the medication for another indication than originally intended. In fact, corticosteroids, which have been used for decades for the treatment of hemangiomas of infancy are not FDA approved for this indication.

Most generic drugs are equivalent to the name-brand product. The prescription will notate if a generic equivalent is suitable.

97. What are the long-term implications for my child's health?

This is a very difficult question to answer in a general way, as it depends on the type of vascular anomaly and if there are any medical issues. It is best to discuss this concern directly with the treating physician.

In general, it is most important to establish the appropriate diagnosis so that treatment, if necessary, can be tailored to the disorder. Sometimes there is no specific medication or procedure necessary, yet the patient will be followed closely by several specialists. Bear in mind that most patients have an excellent outcome.

98. Should we be concerned about the issues related to reconstructive/plastic surgery in children?

It is best to at least obtain opinions from physicians who are expert in this field, who see many patients and have published in the medical literature. It is often helpful to speak with families and patients who have undergone similar procedures. Make certain to keep a list of questions to review with the surgeon, and ask to see photographs of outcomes of similar surgeries. More than one procedure may be required to achieve the best result.

Your child's positive self-image is essential. This will require support from family and involvement of medical and surgical experts.

Jeannine says:

We were told from the beginning that our daughter would be facing numerous reconstructive/plastic surgeries to repair the damage that the segmental hemangioma did to her face, but never did we expected for the surgeon to start these surgeries when she was 10 months old! We were told the earlier the better the result. Three years and numerous surgeries later, our daughter looks amazing! Those who knew her then and see her now cannot believe she is the same child, and those who meet her for the first time now say, "Oh, she fell on her face, and has a little boo-boo?" My husband and I smile. She has been through so much, but it was extremely important to us that she be given every opportunity to lead a normal life and grow up feeling good about who she is, not only the girl on the inside, but the girl on the outside, too—the one the world meets first.

99. What are some emergencies seen in patients with vascular anomalies?

Urgent situations in patients with vascular anomalies include threatened vision, ulceration, functional limitation, and pain. A specialist can help determine how urgent these situations are. In general, urgent situations warrant medical therapy and sometimes urgent surgical intervention. Sometimes patients with urgent situations will require admission to the hospital for initial observation and initiation of treatment.

Emergencies that may arise include bleeding, unwanted blood clotting, airway obstruction, seizures, strokes, and potentially life-threatening infections. These problems often require admission to the hospital, often the intensive care unit (ICU), for higher-level intervention and monitoring. When urgent and emergency situations arise, there will no doubt be several specialists who become involved with the acute phase of the problem.

100. Where can I find more information on vascular anomalies?

There are advantages and disadvantages to searching the Internet. Your physician and other healthcare professionals can help you sift through Web sites and recommend those that are the most reliable and pertinent to you or your child's situation. Listed in the Appendix is a sampling of reliable and educational Internet resources focusing on vascular malformations, which may help direct you to vascular anomalies centers and provide helpful and reliable resources.

In general, however, the Internet sites are divided into disease-specific sites, support groups, chat forums, government sites such as the National Institutes of Health, foundations, and specific hospital programs. So many options can be overwhelming and may lead to unnecessary anxiety. It is best to seek advice from a medical professional who can direct you to the appropriate Internet locations.

You may find it helpful to refer to the listing of references of patient support organizations in the Appendix. Included are listings of patient support organizations that are instrumental in providing additional resources and in connecting people with others who share their story. Many patients and families are eager to provide support to patients with similar disorders. Your physician/ healthcare team may also be able to provide you with

Living with Vascular Anomalies

the names of families or patients who have agreed to be available to others. There is no harm in asking. Alternatively, through family support groups and foundations, you may be able to link with patients who have similar diagnoses.

Through the various patient support organizations listed in the Appendix, you may also learn about conferences and meetings that are dedicated to advancing research and awareness of vascular anomalies. A number of meetings are held for patients, families, and/or physicians.

Appendix

Organizations

Hereditary Hemorrhagic Telangiectasia (HHT) Foundation International
P.O. Box 329
Monkton, Maryland 21111
Phone: (410) 357-9932
Email: hhtinfo@hht.org
Web site: www.hht.org
HHT advocacy and support. Includes factual information, research
updates, helpful links, and a newsletter.

Klippel-Trenaunay (KT) Support Group
5404 Dundee Road
Edina, Minnesota 55436
Phone: (952) 925-2596
Email: ktnewmembers@gmail.com
Web site: www.k-t.org
Vascular malformation advocacy and support. Includes factual information
and resources.

Lymphatic Research Foundation
40 Garvies Point Road
Glen Cove, New York 11542
Phone: (516) 625-9675
Email: lrf@lymphaticresearch.org
Web site: www.lymphaticresearch.org
Emphasis on lymphatic research and advocacy. Includes factual information,
resources, newsletter, and a medical journal.

National Lymphedema Network

Latham Square

1611 Telegraph Avenue, Suite 1111

Oakland, California 94612

Phone: 1-800-541-3259 or (510) 208-3200

Email: nln@lymphnet.org

Web site: www.lymphnet.org

Advocacy and support for primary and secondary lymphedema. Includes factual
information, physician and therapy centers, resources, and a newsletter.

National Organization for Rare Diseases

55 Kenosia Avenue

P.O. Box 1968

Danbury, Connecticut 06813

Phone: (203) 744-0100

Email: orphan@rarediseases.org

Web site: www.rarediseases.org

Medical information and parent support contacts.

National Organization of Vascular Anomalies (NOVA)

P.O. Box 38216

Greensboro, North Carolina 27438

Email: admin@mail.novanews.org

Web site: www.novanews.org

Hemangioma and vascular malformation advocacy and support. Includes
physician list, related support services, patient networking, blog sites,
transportation services, etc.

Operation Respect

2 Penn Plaza, 6th Floor

New York, New York 10121

Phone: (212) 904-5243

Email: info@operationrespect.org

Web site: www.dontlaugh.org

Includes information on the anti-bullying initiative, "Don't Laugh at Me,"
as well as professional development workshops and school assembly programs.

Sturge-Weber Foundation

P.O. Box 418

Mt. Freedom, New Jersey 07970

Phone: (973) 895-4445 or 1-800-627-5482

Email: swf@sturge-weber.org

Web site: www.sturge-weber.org

Support and information specific to Sturge-Weber syndrome, including Centers of Excellence, factual information and resources, and research updates. Patient information is available in English and Spanish.

Vascular Birthmarks Foundation

P.O. Box 106

Latham, New York 12110

1-877-VBF-4646

Email: hvbf@aol.com

Web site: www.birthmark.org

Support and advocacy, including factual information, patient networking, physician list, newsletter, transportation, and insurance advocacy resources.

Disease-Specific Information

Arteriovenous malformations of the brain and spinal cord

- American Heart Association
  www.americanheart.org (Search for "AVM.")
- Brain and Spine Foundation
  www.brainandspine.org.uk (Search for "AVM.")

Bannayan-Riley-Ruvalcaba syndrome

- University of Iowa Hospitals and Clinics
  www.uihealthcare.com (Search for "Bannayan-Riley.")

Klippel-Trenaunay syndrome

- Children's Hospital Boston (Search for "Klippel-Trenaunay.")
  www.childrenshospital.org
- Klippel-Trenaunay (KT) Support Group
  www.k-t.org
- National Institute of Neurological Disorders and Stroke (NINDS)
  www.ninds. nih.gov (Search for "Klippel-Trenaunay.")

Lymphatic disorders

- Little Leakers (Lymphangiectasia)
  www.littleleakers.com
- Lymphangiomatosis & Gorham's Disease Alliance (LGDA)
  www.lgdalliance.org

- Lymphedema People
  www.lymphedemapeople.com
- MedlinePlus
  www.medlineplus.gov
- National Lymphedema Network (Search for "overview" and see FAQs.)
  www.lymphnet.org

Proteus syndrome

- Proteus Syndrome Foundation
  www.proteus-syndrome.org
- National Organization for Rare Diseases (NORD)
  www.rarediseases.org (Search for "Proteus Syndrome.")

Rare conditions and diseases

- MedlinePlus (Search for specific terms.)
  www.medlineplus.gov
- National Organization for Rare Diseases (NORD)
  www.rarediseases.org

Sturge-Weber syndrome

- The Hunter Nelson Sturge-Weber Center
  www.sturgeweber.kennedykrieger.org
- National Institute of Neurological Disorders and Stroke (NINDS)
  www.ninds.nih.gov (Search for "Sturge-Weber.")

Patient Assistance Programs

AboutFace International

www.aboutfaceinternational.org
Support organization that facilitates emotional, peer and social support, resources, educational programs and public awareness for people with facial differences.

Air Care Alliance

www.aircareall.org
Humanitarian organization comprised of volunteer pilot members who are dedicated to community service, patient transport, and supporting public service needs including health care.

Exceptional Parent Magazine

www.eparent.com
A magazine for parents of children with special needs.

Forward Face

www.forwardface.org

Support organization designed to help children and their families find immediate support to manage the medical and social effects of facial differences.

Hannah Storm Foundation

www.hannahstormfoundation.org

Advocacy and support organization for children's issues and for families living with vascular birthmarks and their related medical conditions.

Healing the Children

www.healingthechildren.org

Nonprofit organization that helps to secure and provide medical treatment for needy children. Domestic (U.S.) and international programs provide medical service from volunteer health professionals.

Miracle Flights for Kids

www.miracleflights.org

Charitable organization that provides flights for seriously ill children of families who cannot afford transportation to treatment centers in the U.S.

National Association of Hospital Hospitality Houses

www.nahhh.org

Nonprofit organization providing lodging and supportive services to patients with medical emergencies and their families.

National Foundation for Facial Reconstruction

www.nffr.org

Provides treatment and support services for those with craniofacial difference. This organization is the nonprofit arm of
NYU Langone Medical Center's Institute for Reconstructive Plastic Surgery.

NeedyMeds

www.needymeds.org

Provides information on medicine and healthcare assistance programs.

Share A Smile Foundation

www.shareasmilefoundation.org

Assistance organization for children of working parents whose families do not have insurance coverage nor qualify for Medicaid who need surgery at Children's Medical Center of Dallas.

Shriners Hospitals

www.shrinershq.org/Hospitals/Main

Charitable hospitals in which children up to the age of 18 with orthopedic conditions, burns, spinal cord injuries and cleft lip and palate are eligible for admission and care with no financial obligation to patients or families.

Peninsula Medical, Inc. (Lymphedema Alertband)

www.lymphedema.com/alertband.htm

Medical manufacturer that provides a free alertband to any patient making the request.

Insurance Appeals and Resources

Kaiser Family Foundation

www.kff.org

National Association of Insurance Commissioners

www.naic.org

Social Security Online

www.socialsecurity.gov (See links to "disability" or "SSI" for Supplemental Security Income.)

The Sturge-Weber Foundation

www.sturge-weber.org/(Search for "insurance" to find position paper on the necessity of treatment of port wine stains.)

Vascular Birthmarks Foundation

www.birthmark.org (Search "insurance" or follow link to insurance appeal booklet.)

Glossary

Amblyopia: "lazy eye"—poor vision in one eye (rarely both eyes) due to deficient visual stimulation in early childhood, especially infancy; can be caused by 1) astigmatism (the astigmatic eye causes blurry vision, causing the brain to neglect this eye and the unaffected eye becomes dominant, 2) ptosis (the droopy eyelid may cover the pupil and the developing brain does not receive visual input), or 3) strabismus (crossed-eyes, the eye that is more often misaligned develops amblyopia).

Aminocaproic acid (Amicar; Epsilon aminocaproic acid; Tranexamic Acid): Prevents breakdown of blood clots by enzymes; in vascular lesions with Kasabach Merrit Phenomenon, this medication can help reverse the coagulation abnormalities and low platelet count.

Anemia: Low red blood cell count, leading to pallor.

Angiogenesis: Formation and development of new blood vessels.

Angiogram/venogram: A procedure performed by an interventional radiologist. A catheter is inserted into the vessels of interest, and a contrast dye is injected to directly view blood flow in an artery or vein.

Anticoagulant: Medication or drug that prevents blood clotting.

Arteriovenous malformation (AVM): Occur when arteries are directly connected to veins without the normal capillary bed between them to slow down the velocity of blood flow.

Astigmatism: Flattening of the normally round cornea (the clear structure that is in the front of the eye)—can be caused by a drooping eyelid (ptosis), or by pressure upon the eye from an adjacent vascular anomaly. If there is a larger astigmatism in one eye in a young child, amblyopia may develop.

Autosomal: Inherited on non-sex chromosomes.

Autosomal dominant: Inheritance of a gene on a non-sex chromosome (i.e. not the X or Y chromosome) from one parent resulting in disease.

Bannayan-riley-ruvalcaba syndrome: Macrocephaly (enlarged head), non-cancerous fatty masses (lipomas), vascular malformations, intestinal polyps, thyroid disorders, pectus excavatum (caved-in appearing breast bone), hyperextensible joints, proximal muscle abnormalities, and predisposition to breast and thyroid cancers. Male patients have freckles on the penis.

Bleb: A blisterlike small cystic structure; may ooze or bleed.

Bleomycin: Antibiotic medication that may be injected into certain vascular malformations to make them shrink.

Blue rubber bleb nevus syndrome: Condition with raised bluish nodules on the skin and throughout the gastrointestinal tract; may cause bleeding.

Capillary malformation: Dilation of a cluster of small blood vessels (capillaries), which results in a visible reddish/purplish coloring of the skin; also called a port wine stain, it is present at birth.

Cardiology: Branch of medicine dealing with disorders of the heart.

Chorionic villus sampling: Prenatal test used to determine chromosome abnormality or genetic defect in the fetus.

Coagulate: To clot or thicken.

Compartment syndrome: Pressure on another organ, blood vessel, nerve, or other body part within a confined space.

Complete decongestive lymphatic drainage therapy (CDT): Form of physical therapy for lymphedema that involves massage therapy to mobilize lymphatic fluid, followed by wrapping the affected area.

Compression stocking: Therapeutic device used to support the venous and lymphatic system of the leg.

Contralateral: Occurring on the opposite side.

Corticosteroids: Class of steroid drugs often used to treat inflammation, swelling, and/or pain.

Cowden syndrome: Disorder characterized by macrocephaly, hamartomas, skin tag-appearing lesions, thyroid nodules, lipomas (benign fatty lumps) and/or cancers, and vascular malformations.

Debulking: Surgical removal or reduction of the mass of a vascular growth.

Deep venous thrombosis: Blood clot in deep venous system.

Dysplasia: Abnormally formed.

Doxycycline: Antibiotic sometimes used for sclerotherapy of vascular malformations.

Edema: Swelling.

Ela-Max/EMLA (eutectic mixture of local anesthetics): Anesthetic cream that is applied on the skin to prevent pain during medical procedures.

Embolization: Procedure by which a solution is injected into abnormal blood vessels or structures to create an obstruction or clot to close off the veins.

Embryo: Early stages of growth and development in utero.

Enchondroma: Benign tumor of the cartilage.

Endothelial cells: Cells that form blood vessels.

Endothelium: The thin layer of cells lining the interior surface of blood vessels.

Endovascular therapy: Treatment within the vessel via a catheter.

Ethanol: Alcohol, sometimes used for endovascular treatment of vascular malformations.

Fetus: Development after embryo stage and prior to birth.

Flashlamp pulsed dye laser therapy: Laser treatment that improves red color of superficial vascular lesions; may prevent outward growth of early hemangiomas.

Fluroscopy: Medical imaging test that shows a moving x-ray image of a body structure, often during medical procedures such as catheterization.

Focal: Occurring in one location.

Gestation: Duration of growth of embryo and fetus before delivery. In humans full-term gestation is 40 weeks.

Gigantism: Excessive growth.

Glomangiomas: Another name for glomuvenous malformations (GMV).

Glomulin (GLMN): Human gene and its protein, which play an important role in the development of vascular structures.

Glomuvenous malformation (GMV): Venous skin lesions that include vascular smooth muscle cells and glomus cells; can be caused by changes in the glomulin (GLMN) gene and GLUT-1 (glucose-transporter type 1) protein present on the surface of "typical" hemangioma cells and placenta; not present on vascular malformations or RICH/NICH lesions.

Hemangiomatosis: Multiple hemangiomas, generally on the skin and internal organs, notably the liver.

Hematologist: Doctor specializing in treating diseases of the blood and clotting disorders.

Hematology: Study of the blood and blood diseases.

Hepatic: Pertaining to the liver.

Hereditary hemorrhagic telangiectasia: Familial condition with multifocal arteriovenous malformations on mucosal surfaces (nasal passages, lips, gastrointestinal tract) and/or the brain, lungs, and liver.

Histology: Assessment of the cell organization and structure, as seen under the microscope.

Hypertrophy: Enlarged body part.

Hyperthyroidism: Condition of overactive thyroid gland, which can cause high metabolism rate, faster heart rate, and high blood pressure.

Hypothyroidism: Condition of underactive thyroid gland, which can cause slowed metabolism and feelings of low energy.

Immunosuppression: Prevention of the body's natural immune response.

In utero: In the uterus.

Interventional radiology: Specialized branch of radiology that studies and treats disorders of the blood vessels by using catheterization.

Intralesional: Into the lesion; for example, intralesional injection of a medication.

Kaposiform hemangioendothelioma (KHE): Boggy vascular lesion often associated with Kasabach-Merritt phenomenon.

Kasabach-Merritt phenomenon: Term for when a vascular tumor consumes blood products including platelets and clotting factors.

Klippel-Trenaunay syndrome: Vascular malformation syndrome associated with superficial vascular staining, hypertrophy of an extremity, and underlying venous and/or lymphatic malformation.

Lentigines: Freckles.

Leptomeningeal: Referring to the leptomeninges, one of the layers covering the brain.

Lovenox (low-molecular-weight heparin): Agent administered subcutaneously to prevent further blood clots; brand name for Enoxaparin injection.

Lymphangiectasia: Abnormal dilation of lymphatic vessels.

Lymphangitis: Inflammation of lymphatic channels due to infection/inflammation.

Lymphatic malformation (LM): Abnormal growth of channels and vessels that transport clear, protein-rich lymphatic fluid.

Lymphedema: Swelling from blocked lymphatic vessels or lymph node problems.

Lymphoscintigram: Test using a radioactive tracer injected into the feet and visualized over several time points to assess if there is an abnormality of lymphatic drainage.

Macrocephaly: Enlarged head.

Maffucci syndrome: Disorder characterized by multifocal firm asymmetric subcutaneous enchondromas and dyschondroplasia, improper formation of bone in cartilage, and venous, lymphatic, or other vascular anomalies.

Magnetic resonance angiogram (MRA): Special type of MR study focusing on the arterial structure.

Magnetic resonance imaging (MRI): Noninvasive diagnostic test that produces computerized images of internal body structures and tissues by using radio waves.

Magnetic resonance venogram (MRV): Special type of MR study focusing on the venous structures.

Mediport (or Broviac catheter): Indwelling intravenous access device inserted by a surgeon when medications must be administered directly into the vein to avoid tissue damage that would result if the medication were to go outside the vein.

Mosaic condition: Individuals have a blend of affected (carrying a mutation) and unaffected cells.

Multifocal: Occurring in more than one location.

Nevi: Highly pigmented areas of the skin; moles.

NICH: Noninvoluting congenital hemangioma.

Nutritionist: Expert in dietary care.

Osteolysis: Bony destruction.

Patching (occlusion) therapy: Placement of a patch over the unaffected eye in order to strengthen the "lazy" eye.

Perineum: Area between the anus and external genitalia.

PHACES association: Acronym that refers to an association of symptoms that occur in common patterns involving anomalies of the posterior fossa or brain, hemangiomas in a "segmental" distribution, arterial anomalies, cardiac anomalies, eye abnormalities, and sternal or other midline abnormalities.

Phlebolith: Tiny blood clots.

Physiatry: Area of medicine specializing in physical medicine or rehabilitation.

Picibanil (OK-432): Substance used for sclerotherapy of some lymphatic malformations.

Posterior fossa: Area at base of the skull containing brain stem and cerebellum.

Preimplantation genetic testing (PGT): Form of in vitro fertilization whereby fertilized eggs are tested to see if they carry the mutation of interest; only unaffected embryos are implanted.

Propanolol: Beta-blocker type of medication used to treat a number of disorders; sometimes used to treat hemangiomas.

Proptosis: Prominent or bulging eyes; can be due to mass (e.g., hemangioma or vascular malformation) pushing the eyeball forward.

PTEN: *Phosphatase and tensin homolog protein*, a human gene that regulates cell division by preventing cells from dividing too rapidly; also acts as a tumor suppression gene.

PTEN hamartoma tumor syndrome (PHTS): Cluster of clinical findings (see Cowden syndrome and Bannayan-Riley-Ruvalcaba syndrome) associated with PTEN mutation.

Ptosis: Drooping upper or lower eyelid, which is problematic if the pupil is occluded.

RASA-1: RAS p21 protein activator (GTPase activating protein) 1, CMAVM; CM-AVM.

RICH (rapidly involuting congenital hemangioma): Subtype of hemangioma that grows in utero and is large at birth, then gradually improves over time; may have high blood flow.

Sclerotherapy: Injection of a solution into abnormal blood vessels or structures to create an obstruction or clot to close off the vein.

Shunting: Occurs when blood flows directly from arteries to veins without intervening capillaries.

Stridor: Noisy breathing; can be due to hemangioma in airway.

Sturge-Weber syndrome: Medical condition with facial capillary malformation, often associated with seizures and glaucoma.

Glossary

133

Subglottic hemangioma: Hemangioma inside the airway (windpipe), which can gradually grow and interfere with breathing. The sound it makes is called stridor.

Syndrome: Grouping of physical findings and symptoms occurring together distinguishing a specific disorder, disease.

Thrombophilia: Condition of being likely to develop blood clots.

Tissue expander: Implant that allows expansion of tissue to cover reconstructed areas of the body.

Tracheotomy: Procedure to create an airway opening in the event the airway is obstructed, either internally (e.g., by a hemangioma) or externally (from swelling or a mass pressing on the airway).

Trigeminal nerve: Fifth cranial nerve with three major branches, mainly controlling feeling in the face (also controls some movements).

Tufted angioma: Vascular lesion localized to the skin and underlying tissues; may feel "leathery" and be associated with Kasabach-Merritt phenomenon.

Ultrasound: Medical imaging test used to visualize soft tissue by using sound waves.

Vasodilation: Expansion of blood vessels.

Vein of Galen malformation: Structural malformation of an embryonic cerebral vein resulting in high flow arteriovenous shunting of blood—can result in neonatal high-output cardiac failure, stroke, hydrocephalus, and/or neurological deficits.

Venogram: Diagnostic imaging test performed by an interventional radiologist. A catheter is inserted into the vessels of interest, and a contrast dye is injected to directly view blood flow of the venous system.

Venous malformation (VM): Abnormal venous growth.

Vincristine: Type of chemotherapy drug given by injection into a vein (often an indwelling intravenous line such as a mediport or Broviac catheter is required); sometimes used for hemangiomas.

Index

Index

DATE DUE